T0176631

Neurotoxins and Fillers in
Facial Esthetic Surgery

Neurotoxins and Fillers in Facial Esthetic Surgery

Edited by

Bradford M. Towne, DMD

Clinical Associate Professor (retired)
Department of Oral and Maxillofacial Surgery
Boston University Henry M. Goldman School of Dental Medicine
Boston
MA, USA

Pushkar Mehra, BDS, DMD, MS, FACS

Professor and Chair
Department of Oral and Maxillofacial Surgery
Associate Dean, Hospital Affairs
Boston University Henry M. Goldman School of Dental Medicine
Boston
MA, USA

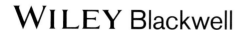

Registered Office
John Wiley & Sons, Inc., 111 River Street, Hoboken, NJ 07030, USA

Editorial Office
111 River Street, Hoboken, NJ 07030, USA

For details of our global editorial offices, customer services, and more information about Wiley products visit us at www.wiley.com.

Library of Congress Cataloging-in-Publication Data
Names: Towne, Bradford M., editor. | Mehra, Pushkar, editor.
Title: Neurotoxins and fillers in facial esthetic surgery / edited by Bradford M Towne, Pushkar Mehra.
Description: Hoboken, NJ : Wiley-Blackwell, 2019. | Includes bibliographical references and index. |
Identifiers: LCCN 2018044565 (print) | LCCN 2018045695 (ebook) | ISBN 9781119294283 (Adobe PDF) |
    ISBN 9781119294290 (ePub) | ISBN 9781119294276 (paperback)
Subjects: | MESH: Face–surgery | Cosmetic Techniques | Botulinum Toxins, Type A–therapeutic use |
    Dermal Fillers–therapeutic use | Durapatite–therapeutic use | Injections–methods
Classification: LCC RD523 (ebook) | LCC RD523 (print) | NLM WE 705 | DDC 617.5/2059–dc23
LC record available at https://lccn.loc.gov/2018044565

Cover Design: Wiley
Cover Images: © Bradford M. Towne

Set in 10/12pt Warnock by SPi Global, Pondicherry, India
Printed and bound in Singapore by Markono Print Media Pte Ltd

10 9 8 7 6 5 4 3 2 1

This book is dedicated to the following individuals:

My wife, whose friendship, love, and support has allowed me to pursue my passion for Oral and Maxillofacial Surgery for so many years. My success would have not been possible without her at my side offering critiques when needed and encouragement always. She has always helped me balance my professional life with my home life and kept me grounded. To my very first oral surgery mentor, Dr. Gary Jeffrey. He was an outstanding teacher, surgeon, and role model. To my former partners in private practice for their support and encouragement throughout my career in private practice. To my colleagues, residents, and students at Boston University Henry M. Goldman School of Dental Medicine who have enriched my professional life. Finally, to my co-editor and friend, Pushkar Mehra, who brought me into academia. These years have allowed me to complete the circle of my career from student to teacher. It has been such a pleasure to work with you and learn from you.

Bradford M. Towne

My father, Mahendra, and my mother, Sheila, for their unconditional love, constant encouragement, and for guiding me to do what is right. To my wife and best friend, Deepika, who has endured the life of an academic surgeon's spouse—I am eternally grateful for the numerous sacrifices you have made to raise our daughter, your never-ending support, and you are responsible for making me a better human being. To, my beautiful daughter, Zaara, who is the shining light of my life, for sharing her father with others. To all my residents, students, and colleagues—I have, and continue to learn so much from each one of you. To my fellow editor and friend, Brad Towne—thank you for your hard work, commitment, and dedication, all of which made this project possible.

Pushkar Mehra

Contents

List of Contributors   *xi*
Foreword   *xiii*
About the Companion Website   *xv*

1   Facial Anatomy and Patient Evaluation   *1*
    Timothy Osborn and Bradford M. Towne
1.1   Facial Anatomy   *1*
1.2   Anatomy of Facial Skin   *1*
1.3   Anatomy of the Superficial Fat Compartments   *2*
1.4   Anatomy of the Facial Fasciae   *3*
1.5   Anatomy of the Facial Mimetic Muscles   *5*
1.6   Anatomy of the Deep Facial Fat Compartments   *7*
1.7   Anatomy of the Ligamentous Structures (Retaining Ligaments) of the Face   *8*
1.8   The Blood Supply of the Face   *10*
1.9   The Aging Face   *10*
1.10   Patient Selection, Assessment, Records   *13*
1.11   Patient Selection and Assessment   *14*
1.12   Treatment Sequencing   *15*
    References   *16*

2   Neurotoxins: The Cosmetic Use of Botulinum Toxin A   *19*
    Jon D. Perenack and Shelly Williamson-Esnard
2.1   Botulinum Neurotoxins Introduction   *19*
2.2   Botulinum Toxins Physiology and Characteristics   *20*
2.3   Manufacturing Process   *20*
2.4   Clinical Usage   *24*
2.4.1   Age of Patient Treated   *25*
2.4.2   Storage and Preparation of BoNTA   *26*
2.4.3   Patient Preparation and General Injection Tips   *28*
2.4.4   Treatment Recommendations for Specific Areas   *30*
2.4.4.1   Glabella   *30*
2.4.4.2   Forehead   *32*
2.4.4.3   Crow's Feet – Lateral Orbital Lines   *32*
2.4.4.4   Indirect Browlift   *35*
2.4.4.5   Correcting Brow Asymmetry   *35*

2.4.4.6   Other Midface Techniques: Bunny Lines   *36*
2.4.4.7   Perioral Modifications with BoNTA   *36*
2.4.4.8   Treatment of Platysmal Bands   *39*
2.5   Treating Facial Asymmetries Secondary to Muscle Paralysis   *41*
2.6   Post-treatment Recommendations and Complications   *41*
2.7   Conclusion   *42*
    References   *43*

3   Cosmetic Fillers   *47*
    Alexandra Radu and Faisal A. Quereshy
3.1   History of Cosmetic Fillers   *47*
3.1.1   Emergence of Autologous Fillers   *48*
3.1.2   Emergence of Non-autologous Fillers   *48*
3.1.2.1   Silicones   *49*
3.1.2.2   Bovine Collagen   *49*
3.1.2.3   Porcine Collagen   *49*
3.1.2.4   Polymethylmethacrylate (PMMA)   *49*
3.1.2.5   Hyaluronic Acid   *50*
3.1.2.6   Dextran Beads in Hyaluronic Acid   *50*
3.1.2.7   Poly-L-lactic Acid   *50*
3.1.2.8   Calcium Hydroxylapatite   *50*
3.1.2.9   Polyvinyl Microspheres Suspended in Polyacrylamide   *51*
3.1.2.10   Polytetrafluoroethylene (PTFE)   *51*
3.1.2.11   Polyoxyethylene and Polyoxypropylene   *51*
3.2   Classification   *51*
3.2.1   Biodegradable Facial Fillers   *51*
3.2.2   Autologous and Allogeneic Facial Fillers   *51*
3.2.3   Xenograft Facial Fillers   *53*
3.2.4   Synthetic Facial Fillers   *53*
3.2.5   Nonbiodegradable Facial Fillers   *53*
3.3   Ease of Use   *53*
3.4   Benefits   *55*
3.5   Complications   *58*
    References   *61*

4   Hyaluronic Acid Dermal Fillers   *63*
    Tirbod Fattahi and Salam Salman
4.1   Introduction   *63*
4.2   Hyaluronic Acid   *63*
4.3   Available Products   *64*
4.4   Clinical Indications   *64*
4.5   Injection Techniques   *64*
4.6   Selection Process   *65*
4.7   Reversibility of HA Fillers   *65*
4.8   Clinical Scenarios   *66*
4.8.1   Nasolabial Grooves   *66*
4.8.2   Lips   *66*
4.8.3   Tear Troughs   *66*

4.8.4   Glabella   *67*
4.9   Post-Injection Instructions   *68*
4.10   Longevity of HA Fillers   *68*
4.11   Conclusion   *69*
         References   *69*

5   Radiesse™ Calcium Hydroxylapatite Injectable Filler   *71*
         Nikita Gupta, Onir L. Spiegel, and Jeffrey H. Spiegel
5.1   Treatment in Practice   *72*
         References   *74*

6   Pearls and Pitfalls of Neurotoxins and Facial Fillers   *75*
         Raffi Der Sarkissian
6.1   Pearls and Pitfalls in Neurotoxin Use   *75*
6.2   Neurotoxin Preparation and Storage   *75*
6.3   Choice of Syringes and Needles   *76*
6.4   Basic Injection Principles   *77*
6.5   Specific Injection Pearls Based on Injection Site   *78*
6.5.1   Glabellar Techniques   *78*
6.5.2   Forehead Techniques   *80*
6.5.3   Periorbital Techniques   *81*
6.5.4   Treatment of Bunny Lines   *83*
6.5.5   Depressor Anguli Oris Techniques   *83*
6.5.6   Perioral Techniques   *83*
6.5.7   Levator Labii Superioris alaeque Nasi   *84*
6.5.8   Techniques for Chin Dimpling   *85*
6.5.9   Treatment of Platysmal Bands   *85*
6.5.10   Treatment for Masseter Hypertrophy   *86*
6.6   Neurotoxin Complications   *87*
6.7   Cosmetic Facial Fillers: Pearls and Pitfalls   *88*
6.8   Technical Pearls   *91*
6.9   Needles vs. Cannulas   *92*
6.10   Specific Injection Pearls   *92*
6.10.1   Fine Lines   *92*
6.10.2   Melolabial Groove   *92*
6.10.3   Labiomandibular Groove   *93*
6.10.4   Pre Jowl Sulcus   *93*
6.10.5   Labiomental Groove   *93*
6.10.6   Midface Volumization   *94*
6.10.7   Temporal Hollows   *96*
6.10.8   Lips   *97*
6.10.9   Nasojugal Groove   *97*
6.11   Complications of Facial Fillers   *99*
6.11.1   Bruising   *99*
6.11.2   Nodules   *99*
6.11.3   Overcorrection   *99*
6.11.4   Tyndall Effect   *100*
6.11.5   Calcium Hydroxylapatite   *100*

6.11.6   Sculptra   *100*
6.11.7   Granuloma Formation   *100*
6.11.8   Vascular Compromise   *100*
    References   *102*

7   Building Your Practice   *103*
    Jay R. Levine
7.1   Internet Marketing: *What's in it for you?*   103
7.2   Promoting Your Practice: Formulating a Strategy   *103*
7.3   Website Design Companies   *104*
7.4   Building Your Brand   *104*
7.5   Print Marketing   *104*
7.6   Website Design: Choosing a Designer   *104*
7.6.1   Other Items to Consider when Choosing a Website Designer   *105*
7.6.2   Designing Your Website   *106*
7.6.2.1   Connect with the User   *106*
7.6.2.2   Outside Perspective   *106*
7.6.2.3   Accuracy   *106*
7.6.2.4   Doctor Bios – How Important Are They?   *106*
7.6.2.5   Accessibility   *106*
7.6.2.6   Additional Features   *107*
7.6.3   SEO: More on Search Engines   *107*
7.6.3.1   Five Basic SEO Steps you can Take Yourself   *107*
7.6.3.2   Blogging   *108*
7.6.3.3   SEO: When to Call in the Experts   *108*
7.6.4   Online Ads: PPC with Google AdWords   *108*
7.6.4.1   Managing AdWords   *108*
7.6.5   Social Media: Getting Started   *108*
7.6.5.1   The Three Es of Social Marketing   *108*
7.6.5.2   How to Gain Followers   *109*
7.6.5.3   Facebook   *109*
7.6.5.4   Instagram   *109*
7.6.5.5   Twitter   *109*
7.6.5.6   YouTube   *109*
7.6.5.7   Pinterest   *110*
7.6.5.8   LinkedIn   *110*
7.7   Protecting Your Practice Online   *110*
7.8   Internet Marketing: Measuring Your Progress   *110*
7.9   Marketing Is Communication   *110*
    References   *111*

    Index   *113*

List of Contributors

Tirbod Fattahi, DDS, MD, FACS
Associate Professor and Chair
Department of Oral and Maxillofacial
Surgery
University of Florida
Jacksonville
FL, USA

Nikita Gupta, MD
Assistant Professor
Division of Facial Plastic and
Reconstructive Surgery
Department of Otolaryngology – Head
and Neck Surgery
University of Kentucky Medical Center
Lexington, KY, USA

Jay R. Levine
President
PBHS Inc.,
Santa Rosa
CA, USA

Pushkar Mehra, BDS, DMD, MS, FACS
Professor and Chair
Department of Oral and Maxillofacial
Surgery
Associate Dean for Hospital Affairs
Boston University Henry M. Goldman
School of Dental Medicine
Boston, MA, USA

Timothy Osborn, DDS, MD, FACS
Clinical Assistant Professor
Department of Oral and Maxillofacial
Surgery
Boston University, Henry M. Goldman
School of Dental Medicine

Boston, MA, USA
Private Practice, C.M.F.-Cranio-
Maxillofacial Surgery Associates
Boston and Somerville
MA, USA

Jon D. Perenack, MD, DDS
Associate Clinical Professor
Oral and Maxillofacial Surgery
Louisiana State University
New Orleans, and
Surgical and Medical Director
Williamson Cosmetic Center/Perenack
Esthetic Surgery
Baton Rouge, LA, USA

Faisal A. Quereshy, MD, DDS, FACS
Professor
Residency Program Director
Oral and Maxillofacial Surgery
Case Western Reserve University
School of Dental Medicine
Cleveland, OH, USA

Alexandra Radu, DMD, MD
Chief Resident
Oral and Maxillofacial Surgery
Case Western Reserve University
School of Dental Medicine
Cleveland, OH, USA

Salam Salman, DDS, MD
Assistant Professor
Director of the Residency Program,
Department of Oral and Maxillofacial
Surgery
University of Florida
Jacksonville
FL, USA

Raffi Der Sarkissian, MD, FACS
Staff Physician
Boston Facial Plastic Surgery;
Assistant Clinical Professor
Division of Facial Plastic Surgery
Boston University School of Medicine
and
Staff Physician
Division of Facial Plastic Surgery
Massachusetts Eye and Ear Infirmary
Boston, MA, USA

Jeffrey H. Spiegel, MD, FACS
Professor
Chief, Facial Plastic and Reconstructive
Surgery
Boston University School of Medicine
and
The Spiegel Center
Advanced Facial Aesthetics
Newton, MA, USA

Onir L. Spiegel, DDS, PhD
The Spiegel Center
Advanced Facial Aesthetics
Newton, MA, USA

Bradford M. Towne, DMD
Clinical Associate Professor
Department of Oral and Maxillofacial
Surgery
Boston University Henry M. Goldman
School of Dental Medicine
Boston, MA, USA

Shelly Williamson-Esnard, PA-C
National certified Allergan Trainer
Clinical Director
Williamson Cosmetic Center/Perenack
Esthetic Surgery
Baton Rouge, LA, USA

Foreword

Neurotoxins and Facial Fillers are some of the cosmetic procedures most commonly requested by consumers today. These services are provided by many different types of providers. This book is not an exhaustive review of all products and procedures but provides a review of what the authors consider to be the most commonly used products and techniques. Our text provides a review of applied facial anatomy related to neurotoxins and fillers, patient evaluation, the pharmacology of the products, the application of the products involved, and potential complications. Finally, we have included a chapter on how to effectively market your cosmetic services in the world of social media.

This text was the combined effort of many widely recognized authorities in minimally invasive cosmetic procedures. Dr. Mehra and I are most thankful for each of our authors' contributions to this book. We hope that you find the information useful and applicable to your practice.

About the Companion Website

Don't forget to visit the companion website for this book:

www.wiley.com/go/towne/neurotoxins

There you will find valuable material designed to enhance your learning, including:

- Video clips

Scan this QR code to visit the companion website

1

Facial Anatomy and Patient Evaluation

Timothy Osborn[1,2] and Bradford M. Towne[1]

[1] *Department of Oral and Maxillofacial Surgery, Boston University, Henry M. Goldman School of Dental Medicine, Boston, MA, USA*
[2] *Private Practice, C.M.F.-Cranio-Maxillofacial Surgery Associates, Boston and Somerville, MA, USA*

1.1 Facial Anatomy

A comprehensive understanding of facial anatomy is a critical component of any facial esthetic procedure. A comprehensive review of facial anatomy is beyond the scope of this text, and this chapter will focus on regional anatomy as it pertains to minimally invasive rejuvenation. All aging changes manifest in different ways for each individual patient, thus an understanding of the changes pertinent for the individual must be understood when considering patient evaluation, planning, and treatment. Incorporating the anatomic effects of aging into the treatment plan will allow the treating provider to target the specific areas to reverse those signs of aging.

1.2 Anatomy of Facial Skin

The face has a layered structure that is best described from superficial to deep and includes the following: skin, subcutaneous fat, superficial musculo-aponeurotic system (SMAS), deep fat, and deep fascia/periosteum. This architecture is preserved throughout the head and neck, with some areas further subdivided into fascial or fat compartments that will be addressed individually. These different compartments and layers may carry different names as they cross anatomic barriers making nomenclature difficult. A special section of the chapter will focus on these terms and clarify some key relationships.

The skin layer is divided into epidermis and dermis. The epidermis is the outermost layer and contains a continually renewing, keratinizing stratified squamous epithelium. The epidermis is anchored to the underlying dermis by hemidesmosomes and anchoring fibrils at the basement membrane. This dermal–epidermal junction provides the mechanical support to the epidermis and acts as the barrier to chemicals and other substances. Immediately below the epidermis, the dermis is the connective tissue composed of collagen, elastin, ground substance, the pilosebaceous unit, and accommodates a complex neurovascular network.

The dermis gives the skin it's pliability, elasticity, and tensile strength. The dermis is divided into two components: the papillary and reticular dermis. The papillary dermis is the thin layer adjacent to the

Neurotoxins and Fillers in Facial Esthetic Surgery, First Edition. Edited by Bradford M. Towne and Pushkar Mehra.
© 2019 John Wiley & Sons, Inc. Published 2019 by John Wiley & Sons, Inc.
Companion website: www.wiley.com/go/towne/neurotoxins

epidermal papillae and sits atop the thicker reticular dermis. The papillary dermis consists of loose connective tissue, fibroblasts, immunocytes, and a capillary network. The reticular dermis is thicker and is composed of more densely organized collagen (which runs horizontally) and elastin fibers (which are loosely arranged). Variation in the thickness of the dermis is what accounts for regional variation in skin thickness. Ground substance is composed of glycoproteins, proteoglycans, and has a remarkable capacity to hold water.

These different subcutaneous arrangements vary in thickness between individuals of different ages, ethnicities, and lines of demarcation into distinct compartments [1]. There is heterogeneity of the facial fat in these compartments, with each compartment having different adipocyte morphology, and extracellular matrix [2]. These different compositions provide unique and specific mechanical and histiochemical properties yet there is little known about the characteristics of facial fat tissue and how that relates to facial aging.

1.3 Anatomy of the Superficial Fat Compartments

The subcutaneous fat is immediately deep to the dermis and is a discrete anatomic plane superficial to the SMAS. There is also a deeper layer of facial fat below the SMAS that will be discussed separately. The superficial layer of fat, or subcutaneous fat, can be further subdivided into two different arrangements with different microstructures. In the medial and lateral midface, temple, neck, forehead and periorbital areas, the adherence of the underlying structures to the skin is loose and easily separated from the skin [3]. The fat is classified as "structural" with a meshwork of

fibrous septa enveloping lobules of fat cells that act as small pads with specific viscoelastic properties [4]. In the perioral, nasal, and eyebrow regions, there is a stronger linkage between the facial muscles, the collagenous meshwork surrounding the adipocytes, and the skin making any blunt dissection difficult. The collagenous and muscular fibers directly insert into the skin and connect the skin to the underlying muscles of facial expression. The fat is classified as "fibrous" with a meshwork of intermingled collagen and elastic fibers as well as muscle fibers.

The superficial fat compartments are partitioned as distinct anatomic compartments (nasolabial, jowl, cheek, forehead/temporal, and orbital [Figure 1.1]).

The nasolabial fat compartment lies medial to the cheek fat and while separate, overlaps the jowl fat. The orbicularis retaining ligament (ORL) represents the superior border and the lower border of the zygomaticus major and is adherent to this compartment. The jowl fat is adherent to the depressor anguli oris, bound medially by the lip depressors, and inferiorly is a membranous fusion with the platysma muscle in the area of the mandibular-cutaneous ligament [5].

The cheek fat compartments contain three distinct compartments: the medial, middle, and lateral temporal cheek fat. The medial cheek fat is a small compartment lateral to the nasolabial fold (NLF), bordered superiorly by the ORL and lateral orbital compartment, and the jowl fat lies inferior. The middle cheek fat is a larger compartment found anterior and superficial to the parotid gland. At its superior portion, the zygomaticus major is adherent at a confluence of septa corresponding to what has been described as the zygomatic ligament [6]. The lateral temporal-cheek compartment is the most lateral compartment of the cheek fat. This fat lies immediately superficial to the parotid gland and connects the temporal fat to the cervical subcutaneous fat. There

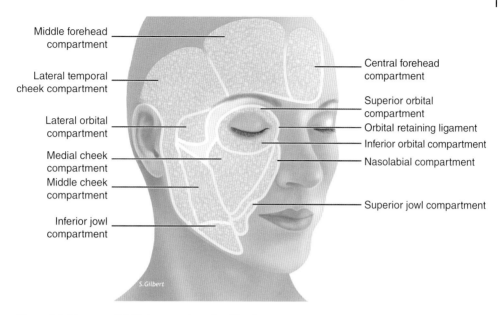

Middle forehead compartment

Lateral temporal cheek compartment

Lateral orbital compartment

Medial cheek compartment

Middle cheek compartment

Inferior jowl compartment

Central forehead compartment

Superior orbital compartment

Orbital retaining ligament

Inferior orbital compartment

Nasolabial compartment

Superior jowl compartment

S.Gilbert

Figure 1.1 The superficial fat compartments of the face.

is an identifiable barrier medially called the lateral cheek septum which is consistent with the subcutaneous extension of the parotid-cutaneous ligament.

The subcutaneous fat of the forehead is composed of three compartments. The central compartment is midline and abuts the nasal dorsum inferiorly, and the middle temporal fat laterally on either side. The middle temporal fat borders the orbicularis retaining ligament inferiorly and the superior temporal line laterally. Just lateral to this is the lateral–temporal cheek fat described earlier.

The orbital fat compartment consists of three compartments around the eye. The most superior compartment is bounded by the orbicularis retaining ligament as it courses around the superior orbit and sits immediately below the middle-temporal fat. The inferior orbital fat lies immediately below the lower lid tarsus and is bound by the lower limb of the orbicularis retaining ligament. The lateral orbital fat lies below the inferior temporal septum, above the superior cheek septum just above the zygomaticus muscle. The lateral orbital fat compartment interdigitates

superiorly and laterally with the lateral temporal cheek fat, and above the middle cheek fat.

1.4 Anatomy of the Facial Fasciae

Explanations of the facial and cervical fasciae are often complex, inconsistent, and very confusing. The concept of the SMAS was first introduced by Mitz and Peyronie, and while it is a discreet anatomic layer surgically, there are many who debate or seek to adequately define the layer [3, 7]. The SMAS is an organized and continuous fibrous network connecting the facial muscles with the dermis and consists of a three-dimensional architecture in two different architectural models as described by Ghassemi. Type 1 is seen in the posterior part of the face and is a meshwork of fibrous septa that envelops lobules of fat cells. The interconnecting fibrous network is anchored to the periosteum or connected to the facial mimetic muscles and has dynamic properties. This morphology

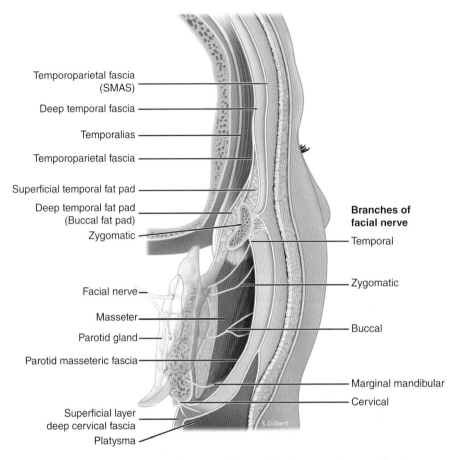

Temporoparietal fascia (SMAS)

Deep temporal fascia

Temporalias

Temporoparietal fascia

Superficial temporal fat pad

Deep temporal fat pad (Buccal fat pad)

Zygomatic

Facial nerve

Masseter

Parotid gland

Parotid masseteric fascia

Superficial layer deep cervical fascia

Platysma

Branches of facial nerve

Temporal

Zygomatic

Buccal

Marginal mandibular

Cervical

S.Gilbert

Figure 1.2 Relationship of the facial fasciae in the lateral cheek/temporal region. The figure demonstrates the complex relationship between the fascia, facial nerve, and the often confusing nomenclature of the continuous layers.

is found in the parotid, zygomatic, infraorbital regions, and just lateral to the nasolabial fold. Type 2 is a meshwork of collagen and elastic fibers intermingled with fat cells and muscle fibers that reach up to the dermis of the skin. This SMAS morphology is found in the upper and lower lip/perioroal region where the action of the facial mimetic muscles has a direct relationship to movements of the lip/perioral skin.

The subcutaneous zone of the face is divided into superficial and deep strata by the facial muscles and superficial fascia which serve as their origin. In the neck, the space of the superficial fascia is occupied by the platysma muscle and it's thin

investing fascia. The SMAS and the temporoparietal fascia serve as the superficial facial fascia of the face (Figure 1.2).

The continuation of the temporoparietal fascia layer medial to the superior temporal line is the galea aponeurotica and fascia investing the forehead musculature. The galea is densely adherent to the overlying dermis with maximal adherence at the transverse forehead rhytids, while the undersurface is separated from the underlying periosteum. Inferiorly, the deep galeal fascia splits to line the deep surface of the frontalis and a deeper layer is adherent to the underlying periosteum over the lower 2–3 cm of the forehead. This fascial construct creates a glide-plane space between the fixation point at the trichion and the lower fusion of the galea to the pericranium such that contraction of the frontalis elevates the brow.

A detailed description of the deep fascial layers of the face and neck are beyond the scope of this chapter, but understanding of the superficial layer of deep cervical fascia is pertinent. This layer of investing fascia is deep to the platysma muscle, continues above the mandible as the parotid-masseteric fascia, above the zygomatic arch as the deep temporal fascia, and above the superior temporal line as the pericranium. During the transit of this deep layer, there are many subdivisions and extensions that invest muscles, transit vessels, nerves, and lymphatics, and create anatomic potential spaces.

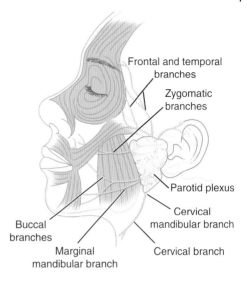

Figure 1.3 The relationship of the facial nerve to the underlying facial musculature.

1.5 Anatomy of the Facial Mimetic Muscles

The facial mimetic muscles are a complex balance of elevators, depressors, abductors, adductors, sphincters, that allow for facial expression, and certain facial functions. These muscles originate from the underlying soft tissues (SMAS) and insert into the skin, not to move the body, but to move the skin and underlying structures. The actions of these muscles assist in mastication, vision, smell, respiration, speech, and communication. These muscles are innervated by the extracranial branches of the facial nerve (Figure 1.3).

It is easiest to discuss the muscles in anatomic groups. In the upper face, it is difficult to demarcate specifically the muscles of facial expression precisely from surface anatomy given the degree of overlap. The frontalis muscle comprises the only muscle responsible for brow elevation, and it forms transverse forehead rhytids. The frontalis originates from the broad galea aponeurotica which anchors on the posterior nuchal line and is fixed to the underlying pericranium of the calvarium.

Activation of the muscle only moves the frontal portion to raise the brow and creates transverse forehead rhytids. This muscle has two halves and extends vertically downward to insert in the dermis at the eyebrow just above the supraorbital rim and glabella. The muscle lies at a uniform depth beneath the skin of the forehead, usually 3–5 mm deep. In the midline, there is no muscle, only a connecting fascial band or aponeurosis separating the two halves. The frontalis is counterbalanced by the glabellar complex (corrugators supercilii, procerus, and depressor supercilii) and orbicularis oculi muscles, all of which serve as the depressors of the brow.

The glabellar muscles consist of the paired corrugator supercilii, depressor supercilii, and the procerus. The corrugators originate from the frontal bone near the superior and medial portions of the orbital rim. They pass through the galea fat pad before penetrating the frontalis and orbicularis to insert in the dermis. There are transverse and oblique heads of the muscle; the transverse head travels superolateral to insert in the dermis above the middle of the eyebrow, and the oblique head terminates in the dermis just medial to the brow. The oblique head acts with the other brow depressors forming oblique rhytids, and the transverse head results in medial brow displacement with accompanying vertical and oblique rhytids. The depressor supercilii originates from the bony prominence near the medial canthus and courses directly upward to insert in the skin of the medial brow. The procerus is a pyramidal muscle that originates in the lower nasal bone and extends vertically and inserts into the skin between the eyebrows merging with the frontalis. It is a depressor and forms a horizontal glabellar rhytid.

The orbicularis oculi muscle is the sphincter muscle encircling the globe and anchoring at the medial and lateral canthi. There are three portions of the muscle: the pretarsal portion which covers the tarsal plate, the palpebral part which covers the eyelid, and the orbital part which overlies the bony elements. The orbital portion is responsible for the sphincteric action of the muscle, and the palpebral portion is involved in the blink reflex.

In the midface, the facial mimetic muscles are deeper and the facial fat compartments limit surface identification of individual muscles. The nasal muscles are the only group of muscles that have clear surface anatomy similar to the forehead. Just below the glabellar complex is the nasalis muscle, with the upper part traveling transversely across the dorsum and vertically down the lateral sides of the nose. Contraction of the transverse head compresses the dorsum, the vertical heads dilate the nares. These muscles will form the "bunny lines" or oblique rhytids of the nasal dorsum. The depressor septi muscle is a muscle that originates in the columella and inserts into the upper lip which will rotate the nasal tip downward and elevate the upper lip.

The elevators of the upper lip are involved in speaking, eating, and the facial expressions of the upper lip. The zygomaticus major inserts at zygomatic body just below the lateral orbital rim and extends medial and inferior to insert into the lateral aspect of the upper lip. The zygomaticus minor is just medial to the zygomaticus major and both act to draw the lateral lip up and back. The principal elevator is the levator labii superioris which originates in the mid-orbit medial to the zygomaticus minor and acts in concert with the levator labii superioris alequea nasi, which originates from the lateral nose. The levator anguli oris (LAO) is a deep muscle originating in the area of the canine fossa and inserts near the commissure to elevate the corner of the mouth. The risorius muscle arises from the lateral cheek and is variably developed and pulls the commissure laterally. The orbicularis oris muscle is the sphincteric muscle of the mouth and consists of superficial and deep parts. The deep layers act as a constrictor and the superficial can bring the lips together and provide expression.

The lower lip depressors act to balance and oppose the elevators of the upper lip. The depressor anguli oris (DAO) arises laterally and inserts into the modiolus along with the orbicularis oris, risorius, and LAC. The DAO serves to depress the commissure and can be seen via surface anatomy as the melomental fold (marionette line). The depressor labii inferioris is medial to, and covered by some DAO fibers on its lateral surface. The depressor labii inferioris passes upward and medial to insert into the skin, mucosa, and orbicularis fibers to depress and evert the lower lip. The mentalis muscle is a paired midline muscle deep to the other depressors and its action serves to elevate and protrude the lower lip. The platysma originates in the neck as a paired muscle that crosses the mandibular border and inserts into the dermis and subcutaneous tissues of the lower lip and chin.

It has been demonstrated that the mimetic muscles of the face are arranged in four layers [8] (Figure 1.4).

The interrelationship of the muscles has treatment implications regarding

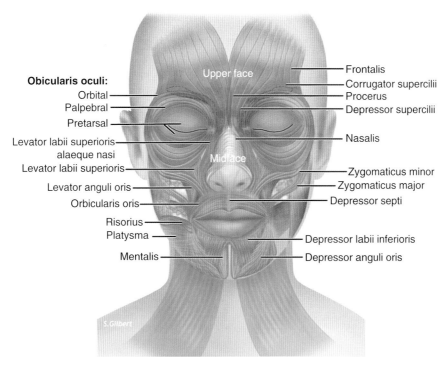

Obicularis oculi:
Orbital
Palpebral
Pretarsal
Levator labii superioris alaeque nasi
Levator labii superioris
Levator anguli oris
Orbicularis oris
Risorius
Platysma
Mentalis

Upper face

Midface

Frontalis
Corrugator supercilii
Procerus
Depressor supercilii
Nasalis
Zygomaticus minor
Zygomaticus major
Depressor septi
Depressor labii inferioris
Depressor anguli oris

S.Gilbert

Figure 1.4 The relative depths of the facial mimetic muscles. The structures in the upper face are generally not overlapping to the degree seen in the lower face. This becomes important with neuromodulator injections as manipulation of lower facial musculature is dependent on depth of injection much more than in the upper face.

depth of injection of neuromodulator, facial reanimation, and understanding the relationship of the facial nerve to surgical dissection. In terms of the facial nerve course, the facial mimetic muscles are innervated from the deep surface in all muscles except for the mentalis, buccinator, and levator anguli oris.

1.6 Anatomy of the Deep Facial Fat Compartments

The deep fat layers (Figure 1.5) are separated from the more superficial fat by the platysma in the neck, SMAS in the midface and temporoparietal fascia in the temporal region. The deep fat layers also separate the deep cervical and facial

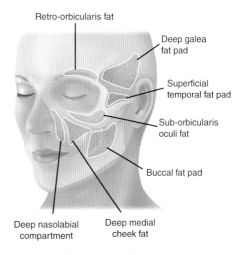

Retro-orbicularis fat
Deep galea fat pad
Superficial temporal fat pad
Sub-orbicularis oculi fat
Buccal fat pad
Deep nasolabial compartment
Deep medial cheek fat

Figure 1.5 The deep facial fat compartments. Evaluation and augmentation of these compartments is critical if volume loss is appreciated on physical examination.

fasciae (superficial layer of deep cervical fascia in the neck, parotid-masseteric fascia in the face, deep temporal fascia in the temple). This layer is separated into compartments by fibrous septae, origins of muscles of facial expression, or bony boundaries.

Several deep fat compartments have been identified by cadaver dissection and imaging [2, 9–11]. The deep medial cheek fat is enclosed by the levator labii superioris alequae nasi (LLSAN) and levator anguli oris, and lies near the infraorbital foramen. It is a triangular structure bordered medially by the facial vein, laterally by the zygomaticus major, and superiorly by the zygomatic ligament. Medial to the deep cheek fat and lateral to the piriform rim is the deep fat space previously named Ristow-space. The deep nasolabial compartment lies superficial to the LLSAN within the premaxillary space but below the orbicularis oculi muscle. Superior to the zygomatic ligament but inferior to the orbital retaining ligament, lateral to the facial vein, and deep to the orbicularis oculi is where the sub-orbicularis oculi fat (SOOF) compartment can be identified. In the supraorbital region, bounded by the supraorbital foramen and extending to the lateral margin of the orbit, the retro-orbicularis fat (ROOF) compartment is located. The deep galea fat pad sits between the deep layers of the galea aponeurotica in the glide-plane space and can joint with or be separated by small septae from the ROOF fat.

There are some discontinuous deeper fat compartments which are superficial to the deep fascia yet deep to the sub-SMAS or deep facial fat. The buccal fat pad is located between the buccinators and masseter muscles and has four extensions. The extensions are buccal, pterygoid, pterygopalatine, and temporal; the temporal extension is continuous with the deep temporal fat pad which lies under the deep temporal fascia (DTF). There is also another fat compartment termed the superficial temporal fat pad, and this is found between the superficial and deep laminae of the deep temporal fascia superior to the zygomatic arch. The superficial lamina of the DTF is continuous with the orbital septum anteriorly, but not the infraorbital periosteum, and thereby provides a space for fat within the prezygomatic space. This compartment is deep to the SOOF and separated from it by the superficial lamina of the DTF [12].

1.7 Anatomy of the Ligamentous Structures (Retaining Ligaments) of the Face

The ligamentous structures of the face consist of true osteocutaneous ligaments, septae, and adhesions; fibrous attachments that originate from the periosteum or deep tissues to insert into the superficial soft tissues or dermis (Figure 1.6).

They act as anchor points, relate the underlying hard tissue of the face to the surface, and separate fascial spaces and compartments. Surgically, these ligaments are addressed to mechanically redrape

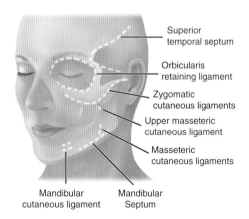

Figure 1.6 The ligamentous structures of the face. These ligaments suspend the soft tissues of the face and can only be altered surgically. Injectables can manipulate the fat compartments of muscles around these points of fixation.

and restore youthful contours. In minimally invasive cosmetic applications, there is no means of alteration, only manipulation of muscle function and compartment volume to restore youthful contours. Understanding the surface anatomy that these ligaments influence allows for manipulation of the underlying structures to enhance the facial esthetic. For example, altering the functional balance between the frontalis and orbicularis oculi with neuromodulators at the lateral orbit allows for brow elevation around the underlying fascial attachments. A consensus of precise terminology, location, and structure is lacking, yet regional description of these structures is relatively consistent. The ligamentous structures of the forehead, temporal, periorbital, cheek, midface, mandible, and neck will be explored in this section.

The zone of fixation in the lateral forehead consists of fusion of the galea, periosteum, and calvarium. At the caudal limb of the zone of fixation, there is a dense fibrous thickening known as the orbicularis-temporal ligament, which is comprised of three ligaments: the superior temporal septum, inferior temporal septum, and supraorbital ligamentous adhesion. The existence of ligaments in the forehead is controversial, but none are widely named or agreed upon. The galea and pericranium fuse 2–3 cm above the supraorbital rim and the supraorbital and supratrochlear neurovascular bundles may act as a retaining ligament lending support to the medial two-thirds of the brow [13].

To describe and refine the facelift procedure, numerous studies have evaluated and described the ligamenouts structures of the midface and periorbital region. In the periorbital region, the orbicularis retaining ligament (ORL) is a circumferential osteocutaneous ligament that originates from the periosteum of the orbital rim, traversing the orbicularis oculi, and inserting into the skin of the lid-cheek junction. The ligament is ill-defined

medially and laterally terminates in an area of fibrous thickening, the lateral orbital thickening, that indirectly connects the ORL to the canthus.

The zygomatic ligaments originate at the inferior border of the zygomatic arch and extend anteriorly to the junction of the arch and body of the zygoma [5, 6]. Zygomatic ligaments have been described more medially along the origins of the upper lip elevators (zygomaticus major and minor, levator labii superioris) though are not as strong as those more posteriorly [12]. McGregor's patch is a variably described structure often used as synonymous with the medial zygomatic ligaments. When described, there was no knowledge of the retaining ligaments of the face or SMAS fusion zones. Anatomically, it is an adherent area over the malar eminence extending from the parotid-masseteric fascia through the malar fat pad into the dermis of the cheek. It serves as a marker for a perforator of the transverse facial artery, the parotid duct, and is superficial to zygomatic branches of the facial nerve [5]. McGregor's patch is an ill-understood structure that should be considered only as it pertains to a historical understanding and benchmark of the amazing strides that have been made.

The masseteric cutaneous ligaments arise from the masseteric fascia overlying the masseter muscle [14]. These are septa that are oriented vertically and form a "T-shaped" intersection with the zygomatic ligaments, with the origin near the zygomaticus major muscle. These ligaments, and the zygomatic ligaments are most tenacious near their intersection [15]. The mandibular ligament is an osteocutaneous ligament that arises from the anterior third of the mandible and inserts directly into the dermis after penetrating the inferior portion of the depressor anguli oris [5, 15]. The parotid cutaneous ligament sits anteroinferior to the tragus in the periauricular area and is oriented vertically. At the inferior aspect of the parotid, the platysma-auricular ligament arises from the parotid fascia anchoring the posterior border of the platysma to the anterior–inferior preauricualr skin [16, 17]. The parotid cutaneous ligament located more superiorly varies in size, density, and configuration depending on the size of the gland, and may interdigitate with the platysma-auricular ligament to form the platysma-auricular fascia [15, 18].

The superficial extent of these ligamentous structures into the dermis allows for zones of fixation and mobility where facial movement takes place. These extensions from the deeper tissues allow for transit of nerves, vessels, lymphatics, and provide a construct that provides stability and minimizes shear. Pessa described these extensions as SMAS fusion zones which are bilaminar membranes that serve as fusion zones between the deep and superficial fascia [19]. These membranes occur at the boundaries between adjacent fat compartments, or between fat compartments and anatomic spaces. This latticework of membranes defines the anatomic boundaries of the fascial spaces as well as the deep and superficial fat compartments of the face. Mapping and identification of the fascial compartments fusion zones is incomplete, though likely to correlate to the fat and fascial compartments that have been described. Clinically, understanding of these compartments facilitates accurate volume augmentation, helps avoid injury to vital structures, and helps provide a structural understanding of facial aging.

1.8 The Blood Supply of the Face

When considering facial reconstruction or facial esthetic surgical procedures such as cervicofacial rhytidectomy, a thorough understanding of the angiosomes of the face is of critical importance as the flap's viability is dependent. Most of the focus and study has been on the arterial supply of the major or named vessels. With the discovery and delineation of the substructure of the compartments of the face, such as the SMAS fusion zones, the arteries, veins, and lymphatics are found to transit these fibrous structures. In minimally invasive cosmetic surgery, the risk of vascular compromise is minimal. The vessels of most concern are the superficial venous structures in the periorbital (crow's feet) and forehead region. These are subcutaneous veins and can lead to significant bruising with needle impingement. Any injection or minimally invasive procedure can also impact the subdermal plexus. The vascular territories subdermal plexus anastomose with one another to form a continuous vascular network, though the transitions are characterized by reduced caliber choke anastomoses. There seem to be three different patterns of subdermal vessels; those arranged in a spoke-like fashion, those with an elliptical skin territory with the vessels arranged in parallel, and those with small and circular skin territory [20]. The orientation of these subdermal zones loosely follows the relaxed skin tension lines, though the implication of the orientation and pattern of angiosomes is unknown.

1.9 The Aging Face

Aging is a perpetual process with an interplay of intrinsic and extrinsic factors, the impact clearly understood, universally applicable and others that are elusive in declaration of their role. Most of the theories of facial aging involve atrophy, deflation, ligamentous laxity, and gravity. There is a genetic component to aging, and while the exact mechanism is unknown, it involves mutations, cumulative DNA damage, free radical damage, and hormonal changes. Chronic disease, nutritional deficiency, smoking, sun exposure, and other environmental factors also play a role. The ultimate effect of these extrinsic and intrinsic factors lead to the signs of aging including rhytids, pigmentary dyschromia, descent of soft tissues, loss of volume, and atrophy of fat. With increased knowledge of these factors, a paradigm shift has come about; from a two-dimensional focus on lifting and pulling tissue, to a three-dimensional perspective where not only the linear but the volumetric is considered.

In consideration of facial aging, just like facial anatomy, it is helpful to consider the regional and component parts that are affected. Aging of the skin is an important factor in overall facial aging. There is a progressive overall thinning of the epidermis along with cytologic atypia in the epithelium, though no evidence of breakdown of the barrier function of skin [21]. Most changes that lead to the hallmarks of facial aging are in the dermis and dermal–epidermal junction. There is a flattening of the rete ridges from retraction of the epidermal papillae and loss of projection of basal cells into the dermis. This results in a more fragile junction which is less resistant to shearing forces. The main changes are in the dermis with loss of ground substance, elastolysis, and decreased organization of the collagen fibrils. Net effect is a less stretchable, less resilient, lax tissue that is more prone to development of rhytids.

Facial aging results from a combination of soft tissue descent and volumetric deflation [22]. Loss of tissue elasticity combined with repetitive motion from the facial musculature and gravity may cause tissue descent; however, the role of the retaining ligaments is poorly defined with conflicting viewpoints. Some believe that laxity of the retaining ligaments results in laxity and descent of the soft tissues along with the known changes in the soft tissues [6, 16, 23, 24]. Others suggest the ligaments retain their strength and the unsupported soft tissues in the adjacent compartments descends around these points of fixation leading to the bulges and grooves that are the stigma of facial aging [25, 26]. It is widely accepted that the bone undergoes changes with aging that has been described as a clockwise rotation with protrusion at the glabella and retrusion in the midface. The changes in the bone may critically impact the ligamentous support, support of the fat, muscles, and skin.

In the brow and forehead of youth, there should be smooth skin, no static transverse or glabellar rhytids. The ideal brow position is at or just above the supraorbital rim with an arch extending laterally that peaks at the lateral limbus in women, while in men, the brow sits at the supraorbital rim with minimal peak laterally. With aging, there are various patterns of transverse forehead rhytids depending on their pattern of dermal insertion. The brow will descend, typically more lateral than medial. This descent of the lateral brow leads to lateral hooding from descent of the tissues around the lateral orbital thickening/temporal ligamentous adhesion. To prevent lateral hooding from interfering with peripheral vision, some patients will activate the frontalis leading to transverse forehead rhytids, seemingly at rest. In the glabella of youth, there is dynamic action of the glabellar muscles but should be no static rhytids. With aging, there are various patterns of oblique and vertical rhytids at rest and on animation depending on dermal insertion and ability of the muscles to generate force. There are many patterns of corrugator orientation with some being more vertical, some fanning out more laterally; in considering any rejuvenation procedure, it is critical to determine the the orientation of these muscles. The dynamic examination, asking patient to raise and lower will help determine critical aspects of muscle trajectory, point of maximal contraction, and dermal insertion. The same examination technique can help differentiate the confluence between the lateral portion of the frontalis muscle and the orbicularis oculi.

In the periorbital area, the upper eyelid is linked with the position of the forehead and brow. In addition to lateral hooding, descent of the brow leads to redundancy of the upper eyelid skin. The skin of the upper eyelid is very thin and with elastosis and further thinning with age, leads to dermatochalasis and redundant skin. Laxity of the orbital septum in the medial compartment leads to herniation of orbital fat, and laterally can lead to ptosis of the lacrimal gland. There is weakening of the lateral canthus which can lead to downward slanting of the lateral commissure and accentuation of rhytids. Laterally, the periorbital rhytids, or crow's feet, are oriented perpendicular to the orientation of the orbicularis oculi. There are static and dynamic rhytids with aging that radiate from the lateral canthus. Most commonly there are three main lateral rhytids emanating from the canthus directly lateral, just inferior and superior. There is a variable intermingling of the periorbital rhytids superiorly with the lateral frontalis, and inferiorly with the rhytids from the action of the zygomaticus major.

In the lower eyelid, many of the main hallmarks of facial aging are manifest. Aging of the midface involves both ptosis and laxity of skin and muscle, bone remodeling as well as volume loss. The underlying bone remodels with bone loss over the malar prominence and lateral displacement of the infraorbital rim. Over time, there is pseudoherniation of the orbital septum and descent of the orbicularis retaining ligament results in descent of the lower lid-cheek junction. The pseudoherniation of the orbital fat creates a pronounced bulge above the orbital rim coupled with descent of the malar fat away from the orbital rim, both serving to accentuate the nasojugal fold (tear-trough deformity). In addition, descent of the midfacial soft tissues leads to accentuation of the nasolabial fold along with atrophy of the deep medial cheek fat.

Closely tied to the aging midface are the nasolabial folds. The nasolabial fold is a transition from the midface and the upper lip. Above the fold, there is a generous layer of fat that covers the upper lip elevators helping the muscle glide in function, while medial to the fold, there is little subcutaneous fat and dense dermal insertion of muscle. In aging, there is an increase in the depth of the nasolabial fold from decreased tone of the upper lip elevators, dermal atrophy, and osseous recontouring. In addition, ptosis of the midface soft tissues leads to overhang of the tissue since the cheek fat cannot cross the dense dermal adherence, and these factors serve to increase the demarcation and depth of the fold. At the medial aspect of the nasolabial fold in the perinasal area, deflation of deep medial cheek fat with age also contributes to demarcation of the nasolabial fold.

In the perioral region, just like in the forehead, there exists a balance between the elevators and depressors. In the aged state, the depressor action exceeds the elevator acting in concert with fat and muscle atrophy. The commisure of the lips turn down and prominent melolabial folds (marionette lines) develop. There is also a deflation of vermillion volume and increased circumferential rhytids radiating perpendicular to the lips and the orbicularis oculi line of function. The loss of bony support in the mandible and maxilla, as well as alveolar support serve to elongate and deflate the lip further. An edentulous state is a prime example of what the loss of hard tissue support does to the upper lip aesthetically. The chin is also impacted with age and becomes ptotic with dermal atrophy, loss of muscular support, and bony remodeling.

Along the jawline, the youthful appearance shows sharp definition of the inferior border, a sharp cervicomental angle, and no ptosis or laxity of the platysma. With aging, the jowl fat and deep cheek fat will descend below the inferior border of the mandible.

The appearance of "jowls" occurs highlighting the laxity in the masseteric ligaments and the mandibular cutaneous ligaments as well as fat descent between them. Platysmal banding, decreased definition of the cervicomental angle, dermal changes, and fat deposition are the hallmarks of aging in the neck. Figure 1.7 demonstrates the hallmark areas of facial aging compared to a youthful appearance.

Reversing or masking the signs of facial aging are the goal of any facial esthetic procedure. A critical appraisal and understanding is the crux of any plan to combat facial aging. Reviewing the literature on aging and our means of treating it has shown a paradigm shift from skin tightening, to volume augmentation. The most encouraging aspect is the intensive study and focus on defining and better understanding the underlying structure and structural changes. With better understanding and intelligence, we are better equipped to fight the battle.

1.10 Patient Selection, Assessment, Records

Minimally-invasive procedures (MIPs) such as neurotoxins and facial fillers have changed the landscape of esthetic procedures for facial rejuvenation. By requiring minimal downtime or recovery, more patients are seeking esthetic enhancement, often at a younger age. Many patients are seeking a preventative approach to the permanent sequelae of facial aging with MIPs and thereby avoiding or delaying surgical procedures. The American Society for Aesthetic Plastic Surgery publishes the cosmetic surgery national databank which shows a precipitous rise in nonsurgical vs surgical cosmetic procedures (Figure 1.8).

Ease of use, low complication rates, elimination of allergic potential, and diversity of products for many indications are some of the reasons that account for the dramatic increases. The evolution of these

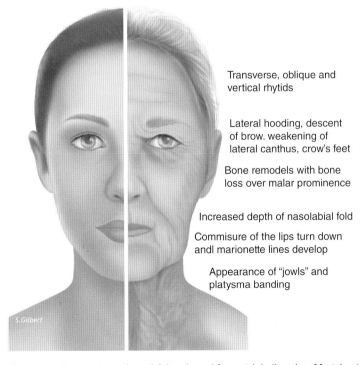

Transverse, oblique and vertical rhytids

Lateral hooding, descent of brow. weakening of lateral canthus, crow's feet

Bone remodels with bone loss over malar prominence

Increased depth of nasolabial fold

Commisure of the lips turn down andl marionette lines develop

Appearance of "jowls" and platysma banding

S.Gilbert

Figure 1.7 Comparison of youthful and aged face with hallmarks of facial aging.

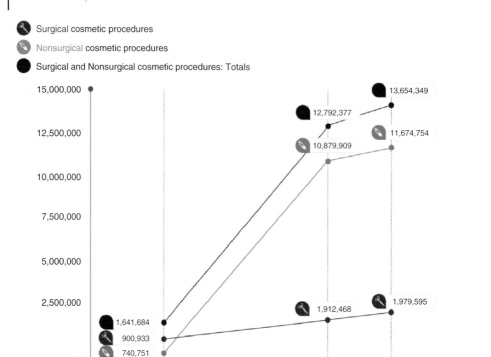

Figure 1.8 Surgical and nonsurgical cosmetic procedures from national databank on cosmetic procedures. Note the precipitous increase in the number of nonsurgical procedures. This includes all cosmetic procedures and further data on facial specific procedures can be viewed through the American Society for Aesthetic Plastic Surgery, www.surgery.org.

procedures has made available esthetic benefits for patients who would never consider having surgical procedures.

Clinicians that provide their patients with cosmetic neurotoxins and soft tissue fillers must have a detailed understanding of facial anatomy and the mechanics of the muscles of facial expression. A thorough appreciation of the aging process including the physiologic changes that occur to skin, subcutaneous tissues and muscles of the face is critical to successfully treating cosmetic patients. This knowledge must be combined with an in-depth understanding of the pharmacology and working properties of the products to be used to restore facial volume. The clinicians must also have an appreciation for the artistic qualities of human facial form to be successful in creating an aesthetically pleasing result for their patient.

1.11 Patient Selection and Assessment

Patient motivation for seeking MIPs varies tremendously but can be divided into three primary motivators. Young patients, generally 18–35, are usually motivated by the desire to augment an area of their face they feel is deficient or prevent formation of wrinkles. The 35–55 age group is usually seeking rejuvenation and those 55+ are usually looking for restoration. These patients are looking for quick procedures with minimal risk, no down time and rapid results. As with all esthetic procedures, a critical assessment by the provider of realistic expectations or pathologic self-assessment is critical.

A systematic approach to patient selection is a critical component of the process. Though there are few contraindications

Table 1.1 Glogau classification of photo aging and wrinkles.

Group	Classification	Typical Age	Description	Skin Characteristics
I	Mild	28–35	No wrinkles	Early photo aging: mild pigment changes, no keratosis, minimal wrinkles, minimal or no makeup
II	Moderate	35–50	Wrinkles in motion (dynamic rhytids)	Early to Moderate photo aging: Early brown spots visible, keratosis palpable but not visible, parallel smile lines begin to appear, wears some foundation
III	Advanced	50–65	Wrinkles at rest (static rhytids)	Advanced photo aging: Obvious discolorations, visible capillaries (telangiectasia), visible keratosis, wears heavier foundation always
IV	Severe	60–75	Only wrinkles	Severe photo aging: Yellow-gray skin color, prior skin malignancies, wrinkles throughout – no normal skin, cannot wear makeup because it cakes and cracks

for MIPs, the appropriateness of the patient for the procedure from a general health standpoint must be evaluated. The patient's chief complaint is assessed in a variety of ways, most simply by asking them "what has brought you in for an evaluation?" A systematic facial evaluation is then performed utilizing a comprehensive database including Glogau classification, assessment of facial thirds, fifths, and a description of any pertinent findings related to facial aging. (Table 1.1). The details from the database and the specific areas affected by facial aging can then be coupled that with what the patient describes as their chief concern. It is helpful to show the patient the areas that you both identify as being impacted by aging, defining a common language that can be used in treatment planning.

It is useful in this evaluation to have a frontal facial diagram (Figures 1.9a and b) that the clinician can indicate location of static and dynamic wrinkles, areas of volume loss, redundant or sagging skin and deep folds. Consent should be obtained and pretreatment photos and or videos obtained to demonstrate the areas of concern. Videos are particularly useful in

demonstrating dynamic vs static rhytids. Also, look carefully for preexisting facial asymmetries. This is very important to document so that the patient is made aware of their existence prior to any treatment administration. Once the evaluation is complete, the clinical findings should be reviewed with the patient. Treatment recommendations should be discussed in detail including the rationale, expected result, and potential risks and complications. If different products are available to treat the same problem, the benefits and risks of each should be reviewed.

1.12 Treatment Sequencing

Treatment sequencing is based on the products to be used and the areas to be treated and will be discussed in greater detail in the remainder of the textbook. Generally, treatment should begin with neurotoxins followed by facial fillers. Neurotoxin injection is typically in the upper third of the face, facial fillers in the lower two-thirds, except for the area of the lateral eye (crow's feet). Provider

(a)

(b)

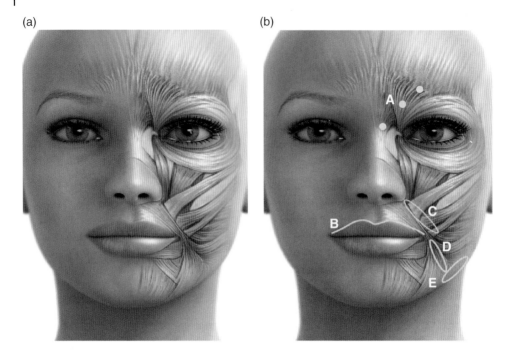

Figure 1.9 This diagram, available from Allergan for providers enrolled in their web site, is a useful teaching and treatment planning tool. The clinician can show the patient the areas to be treated and draw out the treatment solution being recommended. The individual muscles to be treated with neurotoxin can be identified along with the injection sites. For fillers, the area to be treated can be highlighted along with the planned injection patterns. It can also be used as an aid in recording treatment sites and amounts. Figure 1.9(a) Anatomical treatment planning and record keeping illustration. Figure 1.9(b) (A)Neurotoxin injection site, (B) upper lip, (C) nasolabial folds, (D) marionette lines and, (E) pre jowl sulcus.

preference and experience along with the patient's anatomy will dictate treatment sequencing. If both are to be injected into the same area it may be best to wait a week after administration of the neurotoxin prior to injecting the fillers. If a muscle is particularly hyperkinetic and the plan is for filler injection in the same area, allowing the neurotoxin to efface some muscle function will lead to less displacement and better contour. When considering filler injection, starting with the midface is often preferred as augmentation of the midface, cheek, and nasolabial folds can lead to a relative elevation of the lower facial tissues and thereby less augmentation is needed. Ultimately, a balanced face is the goal and a thorough understanding of the anatomic sequelae of aging is essential to accomplish this.

References

1 Rohrich, R.J. and Pessa, J.E. (2007). The fat compartments of the face: anatomy and clinical implications for cosmetic surgery. *Plast. Reconstr. Surg.* 119 (7): 2219–2227. discussion 2228–2231.

2 Kruglikov, I., Trujilio, O., Kristen, Q. et al. (2016). The facial adipose tissue: A revision. *Facial Plast Surg.* 32 (6): 671–682.
3 Ghassemi (2003). Anatomy of the SMAS revisited. *Aesthetic Plast. Surg.* 27 (4): 258–264.

4 Bertossi, D. (2015). Classification of fat pad of the third medium of the face. *Aesth. Med.* 1 (3): 103.

5 Furnas, D.W. (1989). The retaining ligaments of the cheek. *Plast. Reconstr. Surg.* 83: 11.

6 Stuzin, J.M., Baker, T.J., and Gordon, H.L. (1992). Therelationship of the superficial and deep facial fascias: Relevance to rhytidectomy and aging. *Plast. Reconstr. Surg.* 89: 441.

7 Mitz, V. and Peyronie, M. (1976). The superficial musculo-aponeurotic system (SMAS) in the parotid and cheek area. *Plast. Reconstr. Surg.* 58: 80–88.

8 Freilinger, G., Gruber, H., Hapapk, W. et al. (1987). Surgical anatomy of the mimic muscle system and the facial nerve: importance for reconstructive and aesthetic surgery. *Plast. Reconstr. Surg.* 80: 686.

9 Rohrich, R.J., Arbique, G.M., Wong, C. et al. (2009). The anatomy of suborbicularis fat: implications for periorbital rejuvenation. *Plast. Reconstr. Surg.* 124 (3): 946–951.

10 Rohrich, R.J., Pessa, J.E., and Ristow, B. (2008). The youthful cheek and the deep medial fat compartment. *Plast. Reconstr. Surg.* 121 (6): 2107–2112.

11 Aiache, A.E. and Ramirez, O.H. (1995). The suborbicularis oculi fat pads: an anatomic and clinical study. *Plast. Reconstr. Surg.* 95 (1): 37–42.

12 Mendelson, B.C., Muzaffar, A.R., and Adams, W.P. Jr. (2002). Surgical anatomy of the midcheek and malar mounds. *Plast. Reconstr. Surg.* 110 (3): 885–896. discussion 897–911.

13 Knize, D.M. (2009). Anatomic concepts for brow lift procedures. *Plast. Reconstr. Surg.* 124 (6): 2118–2126.

14 Stuzin, J.M., Baker, T.J., Gordon, H.L. et al. (1995). Extended SMAS dissection as an approach to midface rejuvenation. *Clin. Plast. Surg.* 22: 295–311.

15 Alghoul, M. and Codner, M.A. (2013). Retaining ligaments of the face:Review of anatomy and clinical applications. *Aesthet. Surg. J.* 33: 769.

16 Ozdemir, R., Kilinç, H., Unlü, R.E. et al. (2002 Sep). Anatomicohistologic study of the retaining ligaments of the face and use in facelift: retaining ligament correction and SMAS plication. *Plast. Reconstr. Surg.* 110 (4): 1134–1147.

17 Rossell-Perry, P. (2013 Feb 06). The zygomatic ligament of the face: a critical review. *OA Anatomy* 1 (1): 3.

18 Mendelon, B. (2009). Facelift anatomy, SMAS retaining ligaments and facial spaces. In: *Aesthetic Plastic Surgery* (ed. S.J. Aston, D.S. Steinbrech and J.L. Walden). London, UK: Saunders Elsevier.

19 Pessa, J.E. (2016). SMAS fusion zones determine the subfascial and subcutaneous anatomy of the human face: Fascial spaces, fat compartments, and models of facial aging. *Aesthet Surg J.* 36 (5): 515–526.

20 Chang, J. (2001). Arterial anatomy of subdermal plexus of the face. *Keio J. Med.* 50: 31.

21 Lavker, R.M., Zheng, P.S., and Dong, G. (1986). Morphology of aged skin. *Dermatol. Clin.* 4 (3): 379.

22 Lambros, V. (2007). Observations on periorbital and midface aging. *Plast. Reconstr. Surg.* 120 (5): 1367–1376.

23 Reece, E.M., Pessa, J.E., and Rohrich, R.J. (2008). The mandibular septum: anatomical observations of the jowls in aging – implications for facial rejuvenation. *Plast. Reconstr. Surg.* 121 (4): 1414–1420.

24 Owsley, J.Q. (1995). Elevation of the malar fat pad superficial to the orbicularis oculi muscle for correction of prominent nasolabial folds. *Clin. Plast. Surg.* 22: 279–293.

25 Warren, R.J., Aston, S.J., and Mendelson, B.C. (2011). Face lift. *Plast. Reconstr. Surg.* 128 (6): 747e–764e.

26 Mendelson, B.C., Freeman, M.E., Wu, W. et al. (2008). Surgical anatomy of the lower face: the premasseter space, the jowl, and the labiomandibular fold. *Aesthetic Plast. Surg.* 32 (2): 185–195.

2

Neurotoxins

The Cosmetic Use of Botulinum Toxin A

Jon D. Perenack[1,2] and Shelly Williamson-Esnard[2]

[1] *Oral and Maxillofacial Surgery, Louisiana State University, New Orleans, LA, USA*
[2] *Williamson Cosmetic Center/Perenack Esthetic Surgery, Baton Rouge, LA, USA*

2.1 Botulinum Neurotoxins Introduction

The cosmetic use of botulinum neurotoxin A has been one of the main revolutionary forces in the cosmetic surgery world over the past 30 years. From its initial description for use to smooth mimetic lines of the upper face in the 1980s, it has grown to become the most commonly performed cosmetic procedure in the world. Its success is easy to understand; the technique is relatively simple to learn and perform, results are predictable, and downtime is minimal. Complications are rare and typically self-limited. Few cosmetic procedures offer so much for the patient and practitioner, with so few negatives.

The effects of botulinum neurotoxins (BoNTs) had been noted as early as the first recognized outbreak of botulism in Wilbad, Germany in 1793. Initially linked to consumption of blood sausage, the illness became known as botulism, based on "botulus," the Latin word for sausage. In 1897 the clinical illness of botulism was eventually linked to an exotoxin, and not an infection, produced by an obligate anaerobic bacterium, *Clostridium botulinum*. Within 50 years two distinct strains (A and B) of the Clostridium bacterium were identified and eventually eight distinct toxic serotypes would be described (A, B, C1, C2, D, E, F, and G). The exotoxins released were found to inhibit acetylcholine (ACh) vesicular neurotransmitter release by interacting with the exocytic release mechanism. At the neuromuscular junction, the clinical effect was to reduce muscular contraction. In other tissues that rely on ACh as a neurotransmitter, the clinical effect was related to the function of the target tissue; decreased sweating from sweat glands, or decreased salivary flow from salivary glands [1].

The medical use of BoNT was studied as early as the 1940s. In the late 1970s, the drug Oculinum, botulinum toxin type A, (BoNTA) was used in studies to evaluate treatment of strabismus and blepharospasm. Observations during the treatment of strabismus noted that while the muscular disorder was improved, the muscular blockade also occasionally extended to the lateral aspect of the orbicularis oculi muscle causing the relaxation of the mimetic "crow's feet" lines. Patients in the study appreciated the softening effect on their "crow's feet lines" and asked for treatment of the opposite non-strabismus eye to make the effect symmetric. Thus, the first

Neurotoxins and Fillers in Facial Esthetic Surgery, First Edition. Edited by Bradford M. Towne and Pushkar Mehra.
© 2019 John Wiley & Sons, Inc. Published 2019 by John Wiley & Sons, Inc.
Companion website: www.wiley.com/go/towne/neurotoxins

cosmetic use of botulinum toxin was performed [1–3].

Subsequent studies led to Food and Drug Administration (FDA) approval in the USA for treatment of numerous medical conditions related to BoNT's ability to locally interfere with the release of acetylcholine. Strabismus and blepharospasm (1989), cervical dystonias (2000), glabellar rhytids (2002), axillary hyperhidrosis (2004), chronic migraine headaches in adults (2010), crow's feet lines (2013), and overactive bladder (2013). Additionally, BoNT is used "off-label" for numerous other conditions including temporomandibular dysfunction (TMD), trigeminal neuralgia, and all other cosmetic uses related to mimetic line treatment, and/or cosmetic muscular weakening effects.

The use of BoNT for cosmetic purposes has continued to grow in the USA year over year with a nearly 6500% increase from 1997 to 2015. The American Society for Aesthetic Plastic Surgery estimates that there were over four million cosmetic BoNT injections performed in the USA during 2015 [4].

2.2 Botulinum Toxins Physiology and Characteristics

While there exist medical grade preparations of both BoNTA and BoNTB in the USA, clinically only BoNTA is used for cosmetic purposes. The active particle in BoNTA preparations is a 150 kDa dichain protein linked by a disulfide bond [5, 6]. After injection into a tissue this particle binds to an ACh producing neuronal endplate (typically at a neuromuscular junction) and is internalized. Once inside the neuron, the neurotoxin proteolytically cleaves the SNAP 25 protein of the Snare complex. This complex is responsible for moving acetylcholine containing vesicles to the neuronal membrane for neurotransmitter release. In muscular tissue, the absence of ACh release results in a

flaccid paralysis of the associated striated muscle. Clinically this results in muscle weakening noticeable within a few days. This muscle weakening progresses until the maximum result is achieved somewhere between two and three weeks post injection [7]. The delay in this final result appears to be due to ACh vesicles that were already bound to the membrane and available for release prior to the internalization of the BoNT. Once these residual vesicles are depleted the maximum effect is reached. This effect on the neuronal endplate is irreversible, however, due to neuronal production of new axonal sprouts, the tissue is reinnervated within three to six months. Clinically this correlates with the duration of the product's efficacy [7–9].

There are three main BoNTA products available in the USA today. OnabotulinumtoxinA, produced by Allergan, Inc., Irvine CA, USA, is marketed as Botox Cosmetic. AbobotulinumtoxinA, produced by Ipsen Ltd, Slough, UK, is marketed as Dysport. IncobotulinumtoxinA, produced by Merz Pharmaceuticals GmbH, Frankfurt am Main, Germany, is marketed as Xeomin [10–13] (Figure 2.1).

While all three BoNTA products block ACh vesicular release, clinical performance of the three show differences related to dose and efficacy. These differences arise from variation of manufacturing processes, formulation, and potency testing methods (Table 2.1). For the clinician attempting to decide which product to use, this creates a confusing decision-making process that is worsened by conflicting scientific studies on the three BoNTA.

2.3 Manufacturing Process

Unlike chemically synthesized drugs, BoNT is a biologic protein complex harvested and purified from a living bacterium. Neurotoxin serotype and protein composition of the

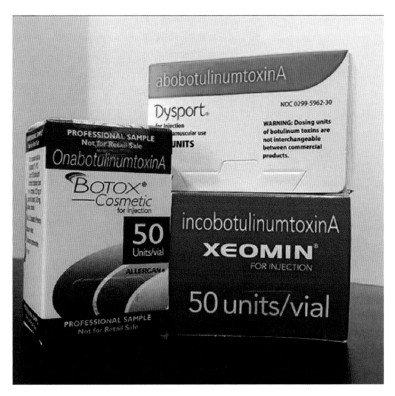

Figure 2.1 Packaging for the three BoNTA products. Note that a 50 unit vial of Botox Cosmetic and Xeomin are pictured. These half-dose vials are often given for staff usage only. The dilution volume should be adjusted by half.

Table 2.1 Comparison of BoNTA products and manufacturing methods.

Manufacturer	Allergan [5, 6, 13, 14]	Ipsen [5, 6, 11, 14]	Merz [5, 6, 10, 14]
Proprietary name	Botox cosmetic	Dysport	Xeomin
Nonproprietary name	OnabotulinumtoxinA	AbobotulinumtoxinA	IncobotulinumtoxinA
Purification Method	Crystallization	Chromatography	Chromatography
Purification product	BoNTA – 900 kDa complex protein	BoNTA complex sizes <500 kDa (exact weights and composition has not been reported by the manufacturer)	150 kDa BoNTA protein only
Excipients	In 100-unit vial: –900 μg NaCl –500 μg human serum albumin	In 500-unit vial: –2.5 mg lactose 125 μg human serum albumin	In 100-unit vial: –4.7 mg sucrose –1 mg human serum albumin
Finishing	Vacuum dried	Freeze dried	Lyophilized

complex is dependent upon the strain of the organism [14, 15]. The manufacturing process to grow the bacterium and isolate the neurotoxin is tightly controlled, as small alterations in technique may lead to large changes in the clinical characteristics of the BoNTA produced. All three commercial bacterium strains produce the 150 kDa neurotoxin particle that is responsible for the BoNT muscle-relaxing effect. The Xeomin product consists only of the 150 kDa particle, while Botox Cosmetic and Dysport also contain neurotoxin accessory proteins (NAPs) of various sizes (300, 500, 900 kDa) depending upon the strain. While associated NAPs theoretically act to help stabilize and protect the 150 kDa particle, research has been inconclusive of their impact on clinical effect [16–18]. The 150 kDa particle must first dissociate from the NAP within the injected tissue to bind to the neuron, but the exact duration of this process is undetermined. Some studies have suggested that at physiologic pH levels the NAPs remain largely associated with the NT, other studies have suggested that NAP dissociation occurs either shortly before or after injection [16, 17], within less than one minute. Clinical studies have shown that all three products will initiate muscle weakness in the target tissue within three to five days after injection. Conflicting studies exist that directly compare one product to another in terms of onset of action but there appears to be no clear difference [7, 18].

Immunogenicity of the 150 kDa particle and NAPs has also been studied. It was initially theorized that NAP-containing BoNTA products would have a greater chance of stimulating an immunogenic response that would in turn neutralize the 150 kDa particle. However, subsequent studies have confirmed that although NAPs may stimulate an immunogenic response, it does not appear to harm the activity of the 150 kDa particle and are non-neutralizing. Preclinical studies have suggested the NAPs may in fact act to protect the 150 kDa particle from stimulating an immune response by physically "hiding" the antigenic portion of the 150 kDa protein from the immune system [19–21]. Clinically, allergic reaction and non-reactivity due to particle inactivation is exceedingly rare with no differences conclusively shown between the three products. Non-reaction after therapeutic injection is far more likely due to other factors such as product storage, handling, preparation, and technique of injection. Additionally, patient satisfaction which correlates highly to efficacy and duration of effect may decrease over time with repeated injections due to muscle compensation in the area, repeated frequent injections resulting in overlapping reinnervation of the muscle, and increased expectations.

Dosing of the three products also creates a dilemma for the practitioner looking to achieve similar results between different products on the same patient. As no international standards exist for measuring potency for BoNT, each manufacturer has its own proprietary method for testing potency units and a product-specific reference standard. Clinically, Botox Cosmetic and Xeomin are supplied in 100 unit vials while Dysport supplies a 300 unit vial. Studies comparing unit dosage equivalency between the three products have yielded conflicting results. In general, 1 unit of Botox Cosmetic is roughly equal to 1 unit of Xeomin, with both equal to 2.5–3 units of Dysport. As a matter of safety the LD50 for Botox Cosmetic in mice is 1 unit. The LD50 for humans is estimated at 2500–3000 units for a 70 kg man, or $40\,U\,kg^{-1}$. Assuming a 25 unit treatment for glabellar lines, this represents a 100-fold margin of safety [6, 10, 11, 13].

Diffusion of BoNTA is also an important consideration when performing an injection. Ideally, the practitioner would be able to target only the intended muscle with no interaction of adjacent musculature. In general, there is little evidence that there exists any difference in diffusion of action between the three products. A number of studies have attempted to quantify diffusion. Injection halo studies use a BoNT injection to block sweating in the underarm area. Starch is applied to the area after maximum effect has been achieved to delineate the area of decreased sweating thereby allowing mapping of diffusion. Difficulties in standardizing dosing and dilution create uncertainty in these studies [22–25]. Clinically, increasing the unit dilution seems to correlate with greater diffusion. BoNTA in standard injection dilution and dosage typically may diffuse in a 1 cm radius from injection delivery point.

Duration of action is physiologically correlated with new axonal sprouting and subsequent reinnervation. However, in clinical practice, the duration of the achieved final result may vary depending upon numerous factors. Practically speaking, most patients do not desire a "frozen" look and wish to maintain some movement in the muscles of facial expression. Treatment thus is aimed at delivering a result somewhere between no movement, "frozen," and total movement, a "nonresult." In general, the closer the patient is treated with little to no movement, the longer the perceived result appears to last. Anecdotally, patients who desire a very mild weakening of a mimetic line, seem to recover movement faster. Similarly, patients who report having a suboptimal result at three weeks post injection often relate a story that the "Botox didn't last" as long as previous treatments. This effect may be due to adjacent untreated muscle recruitment, muscle accommodation or patient perception due to dissatisfaction. On the opposite side of the spectrum, patients requesting the "frozen look" may also occasionally self-report a sense that the treatment didn't last as long as desired, even though the practitioner evaluation evidences a normal efficacy response and duration of three to six months. These

patients often appear for an appointment at two months post treatment requesting BoNTA reinjection at the first sign of subtle movement. One problematic aspect in this scenario relates to patient expectations and perceptions of what is achievable with BoNTA treatment. Patients need to realize that the BoNTA effect gradually wears off somewhere between three and six months, and that sometimes a complete muscle block is not achievable. The other difficulty arises if the clinician agrees to reinject the patient earlier than three to four months. This sets up an unfortunate cycle where the neuronal axon sprouting is on two different schedules, thus requiring retreatment every two months or sooner. This should be avoided as not only does this tend to increase patient dissatisfaction and cost to the patient, but also repeat exposure increases the risk of antibody formation and inactivation of BoNTA. Ideally, these patients should be encouraged to completely allow muscle function to return, then proceed with an appropriate BoNTA treatment.

In comparison studies of clinical duration of efficacy between the three commercially available products, results have been conflicting. The difficulty in these studies arises from the non-interchangeability of the products regarding unit dosing and dilution technique. As previously discussed, all three products are produced and tested in very different proprietary ways, thus they are not exactly "apples to apples." Most clinicians who use multiple BoNTA products in their office tend to adjust their technique and dosing to achieve clinically similar results with similar duration of efficacy [26–29].

Contraindications to treatment with BoNTA are generally the same between the three products. These include a known hypersensitivity to any component of the preparation. All three BoNTA contain human serum albumin, but there is variation in the excipients (NaCl, Lactose, Sucrose) used in each, as well as the presence or absence of NAPs. Patients with systemic neuromuscular diseases must be treated with caution, or not at all, depending upon the severity of their condition to avoid an exaggerated response to BoNTA. Patients being treated with aminoglycoside or spectinomycin antibiotics must also be treated with caution as these medications have been known to potentiate the effects of BoNTA. The most common absolute contraindication to treatment with BoNTA is for women who are pregnant or attempting to become pregnant, and those who are breastfeeding [10, 12, 13].

2.4 Clinical Usage

Patient Consultation for possible cosmetic treatment with BoNTA should be treated in a comprehensive fashion as much as possible. This should include evaluation of skin for actinic changes, vascularity and dyspigmentation, and so on and assessment of facial contour and volume depletion or excess. The face should be assessed for the possible role of cosmetic surgical tightening and repositioning procedures. The patient's expectations and goals should be explored to achieve a consensus of what is hoped to be achieved. We recommend having a large mirror in the consultation room to aid in showing the patient their distinct features and what might be improved with BoNTA treatment (Figure 2.2).

In addition, it is helpful to have available multiple before and after photos of not only BoNTA patients, but also cosmetic skin and surgical patients. There often exists a knowledge gap with patients as to what BoNTA treatment can achieve. Confusion about the difference between BoNTA and facial filler treatments is common in the novice patient. These issues provide an excellent opportunity to discuss a complete treatment plan that may lead to additional services beyond BoNTA treatment. The discussion also serves to "credential" the practitioner and helps assure the patient that they are being

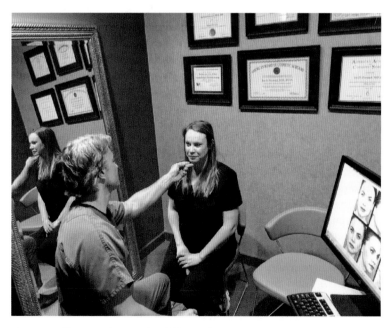

Figure 2.2 The consult room should have a large mirror available, and a computer for displaying before and after photos.

seen by a knowledgeable and caring provider. Even if the patient adamantly wishes to only proceed with BoNTA injection, the consultation provides a platform for proper informed consent and leads to greater patient satisfaction as expectations have been appropriately managed.

Often a patient new to the practice may be seen who has a history of BoNTA treatment and has extensive knowledge of which product and dosing they want. These patients are often resistant to having a comprehensive evaluation and only "want my Botox." However, not uncommonly these patients also exhibit knowledge gaps in various aspects of the treatment and expectations. Patients with previous BoNTA treatment from other providers may have been seen by an individual with a limited cosmetic and surgical knowledge base, and may have received less than optimal information and treatment. Often patients "shop" doctors, looking for either a lower price or better treatment outcomes. All these issues provide an entry point for discussion by the practitioner to credential themselves and better inform the patient.

Most providers find that the initial consultation appointment and first treatment, if performed on the same day, takes about 45 minutes. Subsequent reinjection appointments typically only take 10–15 minutes.

2.4.1 Age of Patient Treated

With the advent of social media and celebrity figures openly discussing cosmetic procedures, BoNTA and filler treatment have become much more acceptable at a younger age. The rationale for treating patients in their young 20s (or earlier) revolves around the attempt to prevent the formation of resting lines in the epidermis and dermis. Indeed, studies of stroke victims and anecdotal observation of BoNTA patients treated from a young age into their late 30s would appear to substantiate the preventative effect of

muscle paralysis on wrinkle formation. Younger patients also sometimes desire to achieve a certain look, or to soften muscular tone to look less angry. ("Resting Angry Face," RAF) These are in fact often the same goals of older patients. While the treatment of patients under the age of 18 with parental consent is legal, it is certainly still controversial. Treatment of patients over the age of 18 should follow the standard protocols of informed consent that one would offer any other aged patient.

While the most common patient age group for cosmetic BoNTA injections is in the 30s and 40s, there is also a large group in their 50s, 60s, and above, desiring treatment [4]. In this older age cohort the practitioner must be cautious of patients possessing a high degree of brow/forehead laxity and ptosis, where BoNTA treatment may be perceived as ineffective. In these cases, the facial rhytids are primarily caused by skin redundancy and folding, and are not improved with muscle relaxation. Often these patients rely on unconscious chronic frontalis activation to lift the brow out of the superior visual field and blockage of the frontalis will lead to an unpleasant sense of brow heaviness and may restrict the superior visual field. The use of BoNTA to treat forehead rhytids is not indicated and a browlift should be performed instead (Figure 2.3).

Interestingly, a well-performed browlift may convert these patients back to being an optimal BoNTA recipient.

Who can provide cosmetic BoNTA treatment varies from state to state and is regulated by the respective state medical, dental and nursing boards as well as state legislation. Dermatologists, plastic surgeons, ENT/facial plastic surgeons, oculoplastic surgeons and oral and maxillofacial surgeons are common providers. Most state medical boards allow any MD or DO licensed physician to provide cosmetic BoNTA treatment regardless of training. It is not uncommon for family

(a)

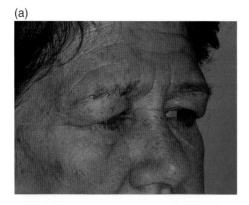

(b)

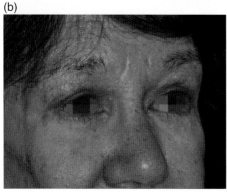

Figure 2.3 (a) This patient has significant browptosis and would not be a good candidate for BoNTA treatment. (b) The same patient after browlift, upper and lower blepharoplasty and laser resurfacing, will now see some benefit for BoNTA treatment of the upper face.

practitioners/emergency medicine doctors to provide BoNTA treatment in medical spas. Physician assistants are regulated by the state medical board and may also be allowed to perform BoNTA treatments with some degree of physician supervision. Depending on state dental board and state legislation, some states allow general dentists to provide treatment. State nursing boards may allow nurse practitioners or registered nurses (RNs) to provide BoNTA, sometimes with or without direct physician supervision. This extreme variation in experience and training among providers gives the facial cosmetic surgeon cause to discuss with patients any previous experiences they had with BoNTA or

other cosmetic services. It is important to always remain complimentary and professional when discussing other providers, but at the same time, any patient misconceptions or untoward experiences should be addressed.

Not uncommonly nurse practitioners or physician assistants may act as physician extenders and provide BoNTA treatment in busy cosmetic practices. For the facial cosmetic surgeon, this has both benefits and disadvantages. While this arrangement frees the surgeon up to have more time for surgery and seeing pre- and post-op patients, it also distances him/her from interacting with the patient on the regular four to six month intervals, as the patient returns for follow-up BoNTA treatment. It is important for the provider team to have clear guidelines on initial evaluation, care protocols, and when referral to the facial surgeon is mandated. It has been the author's experience that the use of physician extenders can provide a non-threatening atmosphere for facial cosmetic surgical procedures to be discussed. Patients who are "not sure" if they want surgery or have a general fear of cosmetic surgery report feeling more comfortable initially discussing the topic with someone they know does not provide the service directly, but is informed. The physician extenders often develop a close relationship with their patients and can add an extra level of credentialing and security when referring them to the facial surgeon.

2.4.2 Storage and Preparation of BoNTA

All three products present from the manufacturer as a scant amount of clear to white powder in the bottom of a small vial. To an untrained eye, the vial may appear empty. Botox Cosmetic comes packaged frozen and is recommended to be kept frozen until reconstitution. In a personal communication with Allergan, representatives suggested that the un-reconstituted product could in fact be kept at room temperature with little to no effect on the product. Functionally, in our office, Botox Cosmetic is kept refrigerated at 2–8°C both before and after reconstitution. It is recommended that Dysport also be refrigerated at 2–8°C after reconstitution. Xeomin alone does not recommend a need for refrigeration of their product, although exposure to extreme heat seems ill-advised. All three manufacturers provide their product as a single dose vial meant to be used on one patient. In practice, this rarely occurs. All three manufacturers recommend the product be fully used within hours of reconstitution, with Xeomin being the longest at 24 hours [10, 11, 13]. Numerous studies have in fact reported little to no change in efficacy if the reconstituted product is kept refrigerated for two weeks. Studies have also shown that refrigeration versus freezing of the product after reconstitution does not change its efficacy [30].

Dilution. When planning to dilute the product, volumes from 1 to 10 ml have been used. Our practice prefers the 2.5cc dilution as this yields a reconstitution such that each 0.1cc conveniently contains 4 units of Botox Cosmetic or Xeomin, or 12 units of Dysport (Figure 2.4).

The argument against reconstitution with smaller volumes is that each drop of liquid may contain several units of BoNTA, and it not uncommon for there to be some "spillage" with each syringe used. The higher concentration thus results in a significant loss of product. Larger volume dilutions mitigate this loss (each drop contains less product), but increased patient discomfort due to tissue distension on injection, and increased risk of unexpected diffusion are disadvantages. The three manufacturers recommend reconstitution with sterile, preservative-free normal saline, in part over concerns that alcohol in the preservative will inactivate the product. However, most practices use a preservative containing saline solution, as it appears to be far more comfortable for

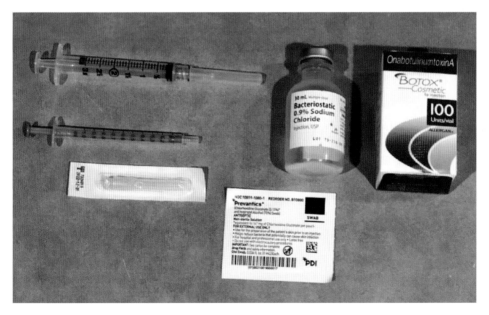

Figure 2.4 Armamentarium required for BoNTA preparation. 1cc Norm-Ject syringes (Air-Tite industries, item A-1) are able to expel all BoNTA solution from the hub, thus saving a great deal of product when considered over multiple patients.

the patient and doesn't clinically affect efficacy. The reconstituted BoNTA solution should be a clear colorless liquid. Discoloration or cloudiness suggest that the product has been compromised and should be discarded [10, 11, 13].

After the practitioner has decided on what areas to treat and the dosage to use on the patient, a 25 g needle is used to release the vacuum in the vial and aspirate the liquid into a 1cc syringe. Example: if the corrugator muscles are to be treated with 20 units of BoNTA, 0.5cc of reconstituted product is drawn up. The author prefers a different syringe for each area to be treated. Once the product is aspirated, the 1cc syringe's 25 g needle is changed to either a ¼ in. 30 or 32 g needle. Sterile technique should be maintained throughout the process. The product is now ready for injection. If the vial still contains product, it is dated and replaced in the refrigerator in its original box so that lot number can be recorded for the next treatment. As the vial approaches empty it is useful to remove the stopper entirely to allow complete aspiration of the remaining liquid.

2.4.3 Patient Preparation and General Injection Tips

The patient should be seated in an upright position. The skin overlying the area to be treated may be prepped with alcohol or Hebiclens, but it must be allowed to fully evaporate/dry prior to beginning the injection (Figure 2.5).

Typically, the patient is asked to animate the area to be treated and the clinician makes note of the presence, pattern, and degree of mimetic rhytids formed. Mimetic rhytids are formed at a 90° angle to the direction of the muscle pull [31] (Figure 2.6).

It is not uncommon for rhytid pattern in the forehead and crow's feet areas to vary greatly between patients (Figure 2.7).

For this reason, we do not recommend that the practitioner have a set dosage amount/fee per treatment area, as this

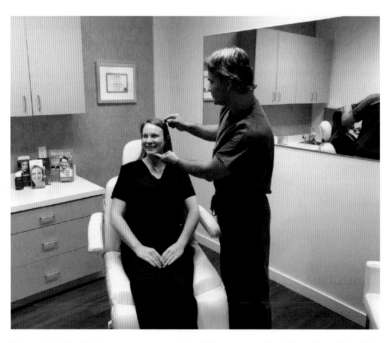

Figure 2.5 The ideal treatment room should have a comfortable, adjustable, chair good lighting, and room to be able to move around the patient.

may result in overtreatment, or more importantly, undertreatment. We recommend that dosage (and resultant fee) should be based upon each individual patient. In planning the injections, it is

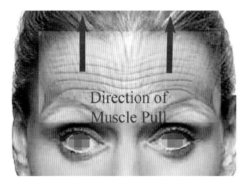

Figure 2.6 Rhytid formation is perpendicular to the direction of muscle contraction.

useful to picture a grid with injection points roughly 1–1.5 cm apart to cover the mimetic lines. Novice injectors may consider marking the patient with an eyebrow pencil in the exact location of where they plan to deposit to product. It is important to keep all depots of BoNTA at least 1 cm away from the superior and lateral orbital rims, to prevent inadvertent diffusion into the orbit, causing muscular blockade of Mueller's muscle and causing upper lid ptosis (Figure 2.8).

Some clinicians prefer to ice the area or spray with ethyl chloride to render the site numb. Ideally the injection should deposit the product intramuscularly. There is no need to touch periosteum and draw back slightly. This older technique often blunted the needle and caused more pain

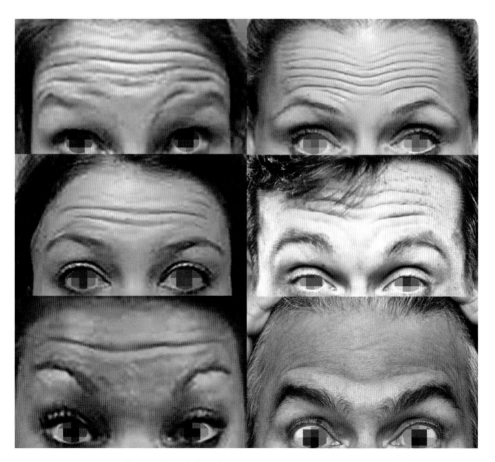

Figure 2.7 Variations in foreheads and rhytid pattern.

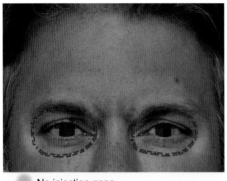

No injection zone
Orbital rim

Figure 2.8 The 1 cm no-inject area superior and lateral to the orbital rim.

and bruising. If the muscle is in a relatively thick tissue, it is helpful to pinch the muscle during animation to ascertain a sense of its depth. Generally, the needle is inserted at a 30–45° angle to the skin. If a pore is in the area of planned insertion, it can be used as an access site for the needle to allow an easier passage into the tissue. It is important to remember that it is where the BoNTA product is deposited as opposed to where the needle breaks the skin, that is important.

2.4.4 Treatment Recommendations for Specific Areas

The upper face accounts for 97% of all cosmetic BoNTA injections performed in the author's practice, and this number is reflected in other practices around the globe. The three primary areas within the upper face treated are the (i) Glabella: the vertical and horizontal lines in the glabellar region due to the corrugators, procerus and medial orbicularis oculi muscles, (ii) Forehead: horizontal rhytids of the forehead due to frontalis action, and (iii) Crow's feet: the lateral radiating lines primarily due to the action of the lateral orbicularis oculi and occasionally small slips of muscle within the temporoparietal fascia (Figure 2.9).

The application of BoNTA treatments for other areas of the midface, lower face, and neck, will be discussed, but consistently these other areas provide a somewhat less dramatic result with more unpredictability. **For the remainder of the discussion, when unit dosage is given, it is approximate for Botox Cosmetic and Xeomin products, for Dysport dosage, the number should be multiplied by 3.**

2.4.4.1 Glabella
The goal of treating the glabella is to decrease the appearance of lines between the brows, and create a less "angry" and more "rested" look to the area. Patients may wish to completely block their ability to frown, or to maintain some movement. The glabellar mimetic lines consist of vertical lines (sometimes 1, 2, or multiple) between the brow, that form when the

A: Frontalis

B: Corrugator

C: Procerus

D: Obicularis oculi

E: Nasalis

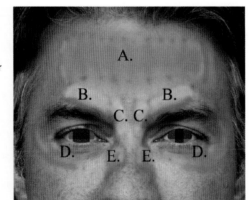

Figure 2.9 Muscles of the upper face commonly treated.

brows are narrowed, and horizontal lines that form when the medial brow is lowered. The horizontal lines present below the vertical lines. While the paired corrugator muscles are primarily responsible for the creation of vertical lines, sometimes called the "11s," and the procerus, depressor supercilii and interdigitations of the frontalis with the medial obicularis oculi are primarily responsible for the horizontal lines, all of these muscles contribute a little to vertical and horizontal line formation.

Typically, five injection depots are appropriate to treat the area. It is important that each depot is at least 1 cm above the superior orbital rim to avoid diffusion causing lid ptosis. It is helpful to have the patient frown and physically pinch the area to find the areas of maximum muscle activity and depth of muscle. The lateral corrugator insertion is into the dermis, and often forms a mild dimple in the skin when active. This dimple sets the lateral border for treatment. In patients with a wide lateral insertion point it may be necessary to use a seven injection technique in order to block the entire corrugator (Figure 2.10).

The injection depots should be placed intramuscularly. The needle should be inserted from inferior to superior to accurately place the depot 1 cm above the superior orbital rim. Each depot is 4–5 units on average, but male patients, and female patients with strong frown activity, may require twice this dosage [7, 9]. Because of this it is important to discuss with the patient their treatment goals. When initially treating a patient for the first time, a standard dose of 20 units for women, or 30 units for men, may be given, but the patient should be made to understand during the consent process that if they are unhappy with the degree of movement at two to three weeks, they would require additional treatment. Ideally, touch-up treatment should be given within two to four weeks after the

(a)

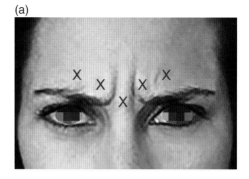

(b)

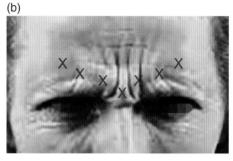

Figure 2.10 (a) Standard 5-point injection pattern for treatment of the glabella. (b) A larger corrugator area to be treated requires a 7-point injection pattern.

initial injection. When patients require a second injection, we make a note of the total units given and recommend this new amount when they present for retreatment in three to six months. Patients will occasionally call one week after treatment with a complaint that the BoNTA treatment has been ineffective, or looks slightly asymmetric. It is important to reassure the patient that the final result has not yet been achieved, and to see them back at the two to three week mark for evaluation. Do not reinject the treatment area at one week. In some patients, it is not possible to completely block all frown activity and this should be discussed with them.

Patient expectations can be unreasonably high when treating the glabellar area. While the goal may be to achieve a smooth, un-creased frown area, often, the repeated movement has caused epidermal and dermal creases to develop. In advanced cases, the subcutaneous fat also becomes atrophic at the depth of the crease. As BoNTA treatment is solely aimed at reducing muscle movement, the patient must be made to understand that this "structural" creasing will not be improved by this modality alone. These residual resting lines may be treated with injectable fillers, fat grafting, and skin resurfacing techniques for optimal results. Before treating the area with a filler, it is optimal to let BoNTA treatment reach its full effect to prevent over-treatment.

2.4.4.2 Forehead

The goal for treating the forehead is to create a flat, smooth forehead that retains some movement on brow elevation, without forming mimetic rhytids. These rhytids are formed by the vertical contraction of the frontalis muscle. Male patients typically prefer more movement, while female patients prefer less, to no movement. Additionally, most females prefer to keep some elevation in their lateral brows on animation, while in men this results in an unnatural, "Vulcan" appearance. Male foreheads/brows should be treated such that they maintain and follow the curvature of the superior orbital rim. Patient goals and expectations are key to developing the proper technique for the patient. Ideally treatment should not result in either a brow drop, or worse, lid ptosis. Brow drop is prevented primarily by assessing how much tone is required by the frontalis to keep the brows in their normal position while not animating. At this point we see the brow position due to the chronic tone of the frontalis muscle. To locate the true relaxed brow position, we like to have the patient close their eyes and relax their brows. Sometimes it is helpful to gently brush the brows downward. This is the true position of the relaxed brows. In patients with a low relaxed position, one should consider either treating the forehead minimally so that some tone is maintained, or considering a browlift procedure. Maintaining a

distance of 1 cm above the superior orbital rim should prevent inadvertent lid ptosis.

The rhytid pattern produced upon elevation of the brows varies from patient to patient. Patients with receding hairlines and a tall forehead may produce considerably more rhytids over a larger area than a patient with a short forehead. Because we expect the BoNTA depot to essentially treat a circle of tissue with a 2 cm diameter, a larger treatment area will result in a higher dosage. Since the frontalis is a thin, flat muscle, the active rhytids can be mapped out on a grid with depots placed 1.5 cm apart. Typically, each depot injection is 2–3 units [7, 9]. Thicker, more muscular foreheads, that form deep rhytids, may require 4–5 units per depot. In female patients, depots placed lateral to the mid-pupillary line, should contain less units to allow some frontalis tone to preserve the lateral arch of the brow (Figure 2.11).

If the glabella and forehead are being treated at the same visit, we recommend treating the glabella first, and then gridding out the forehead injections with consideration to the area of treatment obtained from the glabellar injections. In short foreheads, often only a few depots are required to complete the forehead treatment.

In patients with strong lateral frontalis pull that produces deep rhytids, it is important not to treat only the mid-pupil to mid-pupil center portion of the forehead. If this mistake occurs, it produces a strong, sharp arch to the lateral brow that looks unnatural even in women who desire a higher lateral brow. Small 2 unit depots over the deepest lateral frontalis rhytids will prevent or correct this effect (Figure 2.12).

2.4.4.3 Crow's Feet – Lateral Orbital Lines

The goal of treating the lateral orbital area is primarily to relax the crow's feet lines that radiate perpendicularly to the concentric orbicularis oculi muscle, seen when smiling or squinting. Secondarily,

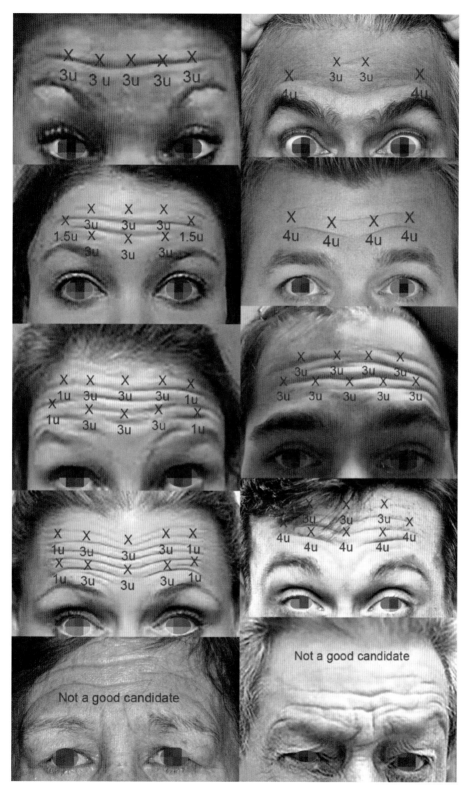

Figure 2.11 Rhytid patterns of the forehead for men and women with the corresponding injection pattern and dose.

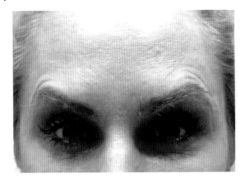

Figure 2.12 This patient's lateral frontalis action has been left untreated, leading to an un-natural "California-arch" appearance.

treatment of the superior-lateral orbicularis acts to indirectly cause brow elevation, by blocking the muscle's depressor action and leaving the unopposed frontalis as an elevator. As with the frontalis and glabellar regions, mimetic rhytid pattern can vary greatly from patient to patient. The depot injection sites can be gridded out, usually 1–1.5 cm apart in a semi-lunar pattern, again avoiding placement within 1 cm of the superior and lateral orbital rims. The orbicularis oculi is a very thin muscle, very superficially positioned, allowing it to be treated with a very superficial injection of smaller depots of 2–4 units [7, 9]. The injector does not need to attempt to "go deep" to inject intramuscularly. Areas of greater muscle activity will require the higher dosage, while peripheral, weaker rhytids can be treated with a 2 unit depot. Some patients will have activation of a small slip of muscle contained within the temporoparietal fascia. Activation on smiling in these patients may cause the crow's feet lines to extend to the temporal tuft. These patients will require treatment of this area and thus will need a higher total number of units (Figure 2.13).

As a general treatment consideration, one of the more common complications in this area is bruising from puncturing one of the many large, superficial veins present. While the possibility of bruising

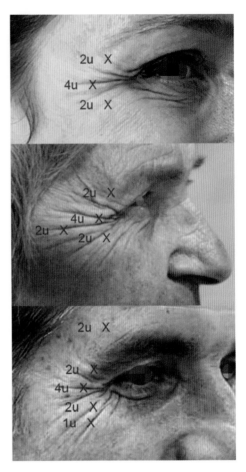

Figure 2.13 Crow's feet patterns and injection locations and doses.

is part of the consent process, this can be a major social inconvenience for the patient. To avoid venous puncture, we prefer to inject, visualizing the area with a low contrast light that allows the blue color of the vein to be more apparent. Use of magnifying loupes may also aid in identification of superficial veins. The superficial injection technique used in this area also helps avoid this complication as the BoNTA depot can be given as a barely subcutaneous weal, thus staying superficial to the veins.

One of the dilemmas in treating this area, is the patient who upon smiling creates an area of strong lateral rhytids extending from the crow's feet, down

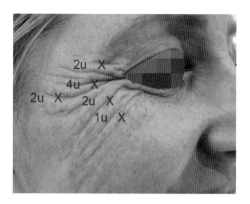

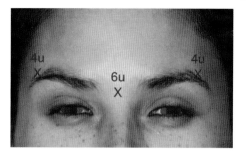

Figure 2.15 Injection points for indirect browlift injection.

Figure 2.14 This patient forms crow's feet rhytids that extend down the lateral cheek and infra-orbital area. Cautious treatment of these areas prevents an un-natural smile or rhytid pattern.

inferiorly to beneath the eye and onto the lower lateral cheek. These lines form due to contraction of the lip elevators (zygo-maticus muscles primarily) and some component of the pretarsal orbicularis in the lower lid. The dilemma is that if only the lateral orbicularis oculi is treated, upon smiling, the zygomaticus' contrac-tion lifts a "shelf" of cheek tissue and rhyt-ids that stops abruptly as it transitions into the smooth lateral orbital area. This creates an appearance that is quite unnat-ural. If the practitioner treats the rhytids below the infraorbital rim to soften the transition, then the risk is blockade of the zygomaticus muscles and a severe altera-tion of the patient's smile. Injection of more than a few units in the pretarsal lower lid orbicularis can result in ectro-pion which is also to be avoided. In these patients, we recommend using small 1–2 unit doses, sparingly, to attempt this feathering effect (Figure 2.14).

Occasionally there are patients who elect not to treat the crow's feet area because this dilemma cannot be resolved.

2.4.4.4 Indirect Browlift

Another variation of this technique is when only lateral elevation of the brow is desired (indirect browlift), but there are no crow's feet rhytids present. This

request often comes from young women in their 20s or 30s. In these cases, it is not necessary to treat the entire area, instead a single injection of 3–5 units is performed bilaterally in the superior/lateral aspect of the orbicularis, usually just under the tail of the brow (Figure 2.15).

This blocks the depressor function, and allows the frontalis to elevate unopposed [32–34]. While this may only produce 1–3 mm of elevation of the lateral brow, it provides a cost-effective and low risk alter-native to a surgical browlift. During an ini-tial consultation, sometimes a patient may only have a "soft" indication for improve-ment with surgical brow lifting. Indirect lifting with BoNTA treatment provides an excellent option.

2.4.4.5 Correcting Brow Asymmetry

It is not uncommon for patients to present with an asymmetric brow height. The lower positioned brow usually will be accompanied by increased pseudo derma-tochalasis compared to the contralateral side. While we think that for large height discrepancies (>3 mm), surgical brow lift-ing provides a superior means to correct brow asymmetry, for smaller differences, or for patients not surgically inclined, minor height adjustment with BoNTA is indicated. In asymmetry cases, it is useful to think of the brow as being suspended between two pulley systems. The frontalis pulls the brow up and the orbicularis pulls it down. BoNTA can be added selectively to either pulley to cause the low brow to elevate, and the higher brow to drop, if desired. To raise the lower brow, we would place 4 units unilaterally as described for indirect brow lift. To drop the higher brow, usually three depots of 2 units are placed in a pyramid pattern just superior to the lateral brow and 1 cm above the rim [32–34]. Overtreatment of the higher brow may lead to an undesirable amount of brow ptosis, so it is recommended that the patient should be seen back at three weeks to assess the results. It is always important during the consent process that the limitations of this technique be explained.

2.4.4.6 Other Midface Techniques: Bunny Lines

Occasionally a patient will report concern over lines that occur on the lateral aspect of the nose when smiling. These lines, sometimes called "bunny lines" are primarily due to contraction of the nasalis muscle, with some small contribution from the levator labii superioris alaeque nasi (LLSAN) muscle. To soften these lines a single depot injection of 3–4 units into each nasalis belly should be sufficient to relax the area [7, 9] (Figure 2.16).

An unintended, and not infrequent, complication of this technique is the likelihood of unintentional blockade of the LLSAN. While this muscle is fairly small, it appears to contribute a great deal to lip elevation during smile. Patients often report a "flattened" smile, that doesn't turn up at the commissures as seen pretreatment. For patients who are insistent to try this procedure it is extremely important to stress the likelihood of this complication. Often, the patient will try the nasalis injection, knowing that it will eventually wear off, but few choose to repeat the procedure.

2.4.4.7 Perioral Modifications with BoNTA

The next four discussions of cosmetic usage for BoNTA target various aspects of the perioral musculature. The ability to phonate, sing, play wind musical instruments, and convey emotion through smiling, pursing of the lips, and so on relies on a delicate balance of interplay between these muscles. For this reason, in all examples, dosages used are quite small, and the goal is only to weaken and not completely paralyze the target muscles. Despite the best efforts of the most experienced injectors, these techniques carry a level of uncertainty and may inadvertently change lip function and animation in an adverse, albeit temporary, fashion. Due to this unpredictability, we do not recommend these procedures for professional musicians who play a wind instrument, or similarly, caution should be taken in treating professional singers or speakers.

2.4.4.7.1 Vertical Lip Lines

As discussed, the upper face (glabella, forehead, crow's feet), is the primary

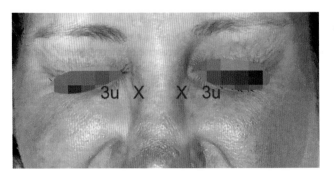

Figure 2.16 Bunny lines and treatment injections.

target for most cosmetic BoNTA treatments, with most other locations offering somewhat less predictability and result. The treatment of vertical lip lines is an exception to this in the right patient. No patient, male or female, ever requests to keep their vertical lip lines if it is possible to erase them. Unlike crow's feet, or frown lines, which can be said to add "character" to a face, there is little beauty found in these little lines. Sometimes called smoker's lines, they can be found in non-smokers and smoker's alike. As with any mimetic wrinkle, over time, an epidermal and dermal crease develops in the upper or lower lips in response to the circumferential puckering of the skin with contraction of the orbicularis oris. These lines deepen and may cross the white roll and vermillion border of the lips and extend radially outward around the mouth. In observing a patients mouth during speech, with very deep lip lines, one is struck by the hyperdynamic contraction of the superficial layer of the orbicularis oris as it inserts into the dermis. Certainly, these patients benefit from moderate and deep ablative and sub-blative resurfacing, and injectable fillers provide the workhorse for recreating lip architecture and filling deep lines. But to correct the hyperfunctioning aspect of the lip animation, treatment with BoNTA is indicated.

Injection technique is quite simple with very small depots of 1–2 units (a drop) placed very superficially, 1–3 mm above the vermillion border, (below the vermillion border in the lower lip) centered over the dynamic lip lines [35–37]. An upper lip rarely is treated with more than 8 units total. Because of the small unit dosage used, the injections are often placed much closer together (5–8 mm) (Figure 2.17).

The lower lip tends to form fewer vertical lines, and more laterally, than the upper lip. It is important to keep dosage low as overtreatment will interfere in normal lip function. Even with appropriate treatment, patients may note that they

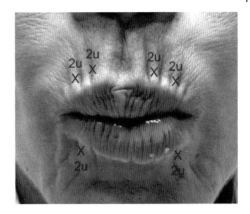

Figure 2.17 Vertical lip line patterns and treatment.

have difficulty sucking through a straw or whistling. Perhaps the most important aspect of offering this treatment is to stress that BoNTA is only treating one aspect of the lip lines, and that they will not entirely disappear. We recommend hyaluronic acid fillers for filling deep lines and reconstituting the white roll and architecture of the lip. This should ideally be performed sometime after the BoNTA has taken effect, but can be done at the same appointment. Skin resurfacing, as mentioned, is effective at smoothing superficial lines that are fine to be filled.

2.4.4.7.2 Excessive Chin Dimpling

Sometimes called peau d'orange, or orange peel skin, because of its appearance, these dimples in the anterior chin arise from the dermal insertions of the paired mentalis muscles. While most people can make these dimples on demand, some patients find them objectionable, or have a chronic mentalis habit and constantly display them. For these individuals, BoNTA treatment is helpful and aimed at blockade of the superficial insertions of the mentalis into the skin, similar to treating vertical lip lines. Each depot injection contains 1–2 units (a drop) and should be injected in a 7–8 mm grid pattern over the area of the chin exhibiting the dimpling [38, 39] (Figure 2.18).

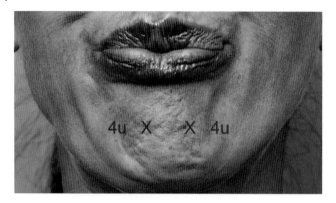

Figure 2.18 Mentalis "peau de l'orange" dimples and treatment.

Deep injections are generally not recommended as they can result in lip incompetence, and difficulty pronouncing the letter "P."

2.4.4.7.3 Downward-turned Commissures of the Mouth

Most patients will display some evidence of downward-turning of the commissures with age. For slight changes, we prefer using an injectable hyaluronic acid to lift and reinforce the commissures. A subset of patients will show an element of hyperactivity in the depressor anguli oris (DAO) muscle that exacerbates the condition. BoNTA treatment is aimed at weakening the DAO symmetrically without effecting the depressor labii inferioris (DLI). A single injection of 2–5 units into each belly of the DAO is recommended [7, 9, 40]. The difficulty with this injection is locating the exact location to inject the DAO. The patient is asked to show their bottom teeth in a maneuver similar to assessing marginal mandibular nerve function. The belly of the DAO can often be palpated in this contracted position (Figure 2.19). This location often correlates to slightly lateral to the commissure and 1 cm above the inferior border of the mandible. One should avoid injecting medial to the commissure as this increases the chance of inadvertent blockade of the DLI. After injection, it is important to see the patient

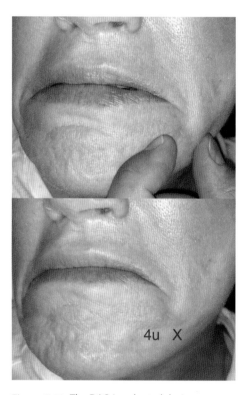

Figure 2.19 The DAO is palpated during activation and injection points.

back within two to three weeks to assess for symmetry of effect. The patient is then asked again to show their bottom teeth. If one side of the lip easily depresses but the other stays elevated, it is the side that is actively depressing that warrants reinjection.

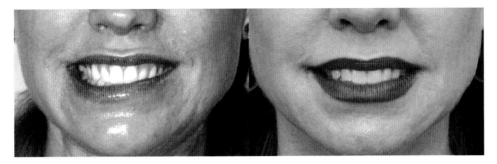

Figure 2.20 An asymmetric injection of the DAO has created this stroke-like effect. Re-treatment of the functioning right DAO corrects this deformity.

Most injectors find this to be one of the more difficult BoNTA techniques to master (Figure 2.20).

2.4.4.7.4 Lip Lengthening

For the patient with a hyperactive, short upper lip, and a resultant "gummy smile", few options exist outside of maxillary LeFort 1 osteotomy with superior repositioning. This technique while mostly effective, often fails to correct the hyperfunctioning lip, is invasive, has prolonged recovery, and is expensive. In addition, short lip patients may have an appropriate maxillary height based on facial thirds, and superior repositioning is not indicated, and may compromise facial esthetics. A conservative option in these instances is to try to selectively blockade some of the muscles causing the hyperactive lip elevation. A number of muscles interdigitate and have a dynamic interplay in this region, and treatment is aimed at injecting as small a dose as possible to achieve a result, while not adversely affecting smile esthetics. The injection technique is quite simple, with 2–3 unit depots injected below each ala and one 2–3 unit depot injected just below the columella intramuscularly [35–37] (Figure 2.21).

If one assumes that the standard 1 cm diffusion radius applies in this region, we would expect that virtually all the lip elevators should be weakened somewhat and the hyperfunctioning lip will relax and drop, and not raise as much upon smile

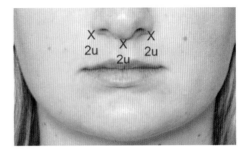

Figure 2.21 Injection sites for lip lengthening.

animation. Similar to bunny line treatment, the goal is usually achieved but smile esthetics may be compromised. It is best to start with a smaller dose depot injection, and increase dosage as needed to find the appropriate compromise in this region.

2.4.4.8 Treatment of Platysmal Bands

Platysmal bands may start to become apparent as early as the late 30s, with almost all individuals having some degree of banding apparent by the 50s. Predictable correction of moderate to severe banding is obtained with platysmaplasty, performed either alone, or in conjunction with a neck lift or facelift. For patients with mild banding, mild recurrent banding after platysmaplasty, or surgery aversion, treatment of platysmal bands with BoNTA can be an effective, if not completely corrective procedure.

Bands that are present at rest are the most common target, but some patients

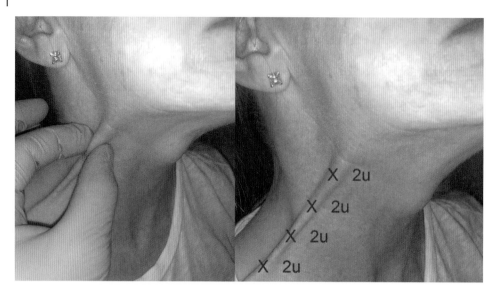

Figure 2.22 The platysmal band is grasped with the non-dominant hand and the injection is given sub-cutaneously or superficially intra-muscularly.

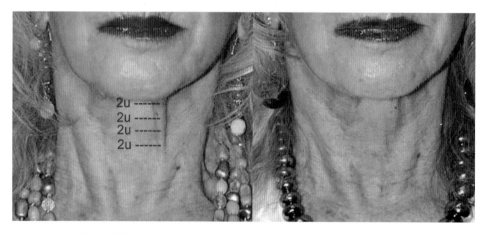

Figure 2.23 Before and three weeks after treatment of platysmal bands.

seek treatment of bands that are only prominent with activation. Because of the close proximity of the swallowing and laryngeal musculature deep to the platysma, injections consist of small, 2–4 unit depots placed superficially along the offending band at 1.5–2 cm intervals. To aid in correct placement, the platysmal band is grasped between the fingers of the non-dominant hand and tented up slightly away from the neck (Figure 2.22).

The injection depot is placed immediately sub-cutaneously instead of intramuscularly.

At most, the author recommends no more than 20 units be used for each side of the neck to limit risk of inadvertent weakening of the deeper neck musculature causing dysphagia, difficulty swallowing, or hoarseness. The patient is seen again at two to three weeks and reinjection can be performed if necessary [41–43] (Figure 2.23).

When treating neck banding with BoNTA it is important to inform the patient of what the product can and won't do. As a muscle relaxing agent, BoNTA only serves to decrease inherent tone in the muscle. This tone is partially responsible for the "cabling" effect as the band crosses the reflex of the neck. One can expect the band to fall back into to the neck contour, but this will not address any areas of skin laxity or adipose accumulation. The technique is particularly useful to the facial surgeon for patients who are three to five years post facelift and some relapse has occurred.

2.5 Treating Facial Asymmetries Secondary to Muscle Paralysis

There are several congenital and acquired causes of asymmetric muscle weakness or paralysis of the face. Treatment with BoNTA allows the practitioner to selectively weaken the normal functioning musculature to create a less obvious asymmetry. Patients with unilateral weakness in the frontal branch or marginal mandibular branch of the facial nerve are particularly good candidates for this camouflage procedure. When planning for treatment, it is important to not weaken the targeted muscle in such a way as to create dysfunction in lip or eyelid competency. Careful discussion with the patient about limitations of the treatment is paramount. It is extremely important that the patient realizes that this is not a reanimation procedure, but rather the exact opposite. The goal is to camouflage the pre-existing paralysis with a matching BoNTA induced weakness on the contralateral side.

2.6 Post-treatment Recommendations and Complications

In practice, there is little post-operative care needed to be performed post injection. In the immediate post-treatment period the most noticeable change is a

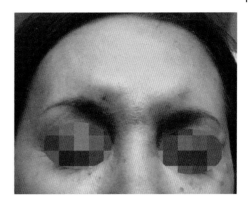

Figure 2.24 Typical wheals present after BoNTA injection.

small wheal under the skin at each injection site (Figure 2.24).

This should subside within half an hour and the patient should be instructed not to rub the area. It is permissible to apply makeup over the area if desired (Figure 2.25).

Occasionally there may local bruising. This will naturally resolve over time, but patients may consider applying topical arnica gel to the area to speed resolution. Ice applied immediately after injection may also limit the extent of the ecchymosis. In addition, patients should consider avoiding any strenuous activity on the day of the injection to decrease the chance of elevated blood pressure exacerbating any ecchymosis. In patients that are known to be on anticoagulants such as aspirin, these can be halted if cleared by the prescribing physician. Small ecchymosis may be due to extravasation from the dermal plexus, but larger areas of bruising usually suggest that a subcutaneous vein has been punctured. Visualization under low contrast light while injecting, and use of loupe magnification can help avoid this problem.

Patients sometimes report having a headache, or stomach discomfort within 24 hours after their first exposure to BoNTA. While this reaction is not well understood, it is considered normal and is should not be too concerning. Interestingly, subsequent treatments rarely cause this problem. Localized tenderness or itching at injection sites is also common and routine [7, 9].

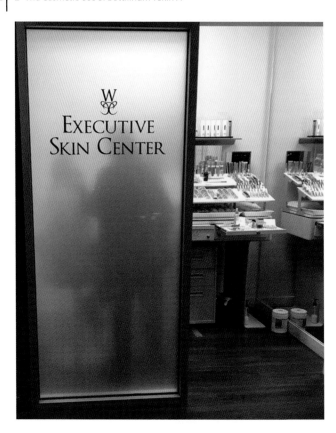

Figure 2.25 Most estheticians are adept make-up artists. This service helps camouflage any bruising.

There is some evidence that instructing the patient to animate repeatedly the muscles targeted for one to two hours post-treatment increases neuronal BoNTA binding and uptake, leading to quicker onset of action and less diffusion. Manufacturers also recommend that the patient stay upright for four hours post-treatment to decrease BoNTA diffusion [44].

Biofilm infection from BoNTA injection is rare but occasionally seen. This typically presents two to four days after treatment as an area of erythema and edema near a single injection site. These localized areas of cellulitis typically resolve with broad spectrum antibiotics targeting normal skin flora.

The most common complication after BoNTA injection, excluding those related to the actual injection, is patient expectations not being met. This emphasizes the need for a thorough pre-treatment consultation and informed consent process prior to initiating therapy.

When treating the upper facial area, the most worrisome complication is inadvertent diffusion of product within the superior orbit with resulting ptosis. Fortunately, this complication is fairly easy to avoid by staying 1 cm outside of the orbital rim. If ptosis does occur, it typically resolves within a few weeks. Iopidine ocular drops can provide temporary resolution of the ptosis if the patient has an important event to attend and is self-conscious of the ptosis (Figure 2.26).

Unfortunately, diffusion in other treatment areas such as the DAO or platysmal bands are irreversible and the patient must be managed until reinnervation can occur.

2.7 Conclusion

Cosmetic treatments with botulinum toxinA continue to be a predictable procedure with dramatic outcomes, little downtime, and few complications. For the

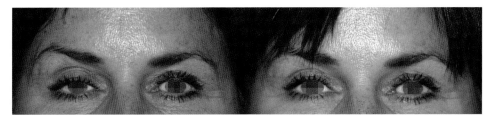

Figure 2.26 Lid ptosis secondary to BoNTA treatment is temporarily corrected with ocular iopidine drops.

practitioner, it is a valuable tool to achieve results for patients that otherwise might be impossible. The numerous possibilities to apply this technology to treat facial asymmetries makes this a truly fun product to use.

References

1 Schantz, E.J. and Johnson, E.A. (1997). Botulinum toxin: the story of its development for the treatment of human disease. *Perspect Biol Med* 40 (3): 317–327.

2 Carruthers, J.D. and Carruthers, J.A. (1992). Treatment of glabellar frown lines with C. Botulinum-a exotoxin. *J Dermatol Surg Oncol* 18: 17–21.

3 Carruthers, A. (2002). Botulinum toxin type a: history and current cosmetic use in the upper face. *Dis Mon* 48: 299–322.

4 American Society for Aesthetic Plastic Surgery. Cosmetic Surgery National Data Bank statistics. American Society for Aesthetic Plastic Surgery website. http://www.surgery.org/sites/default/files/ASAPS-Stats2015.pdf.

5 Hambleton, P. (1992). Clostridium botulinum toxins: a general review of involvement in disease, structure, mode of action and preparation for clinical use. *J Neurol* 239 (1): 16–20.

6 Panjwani, N., O'Keeffe, R., and Pickett, A. (2008). Biochemical, functional and potency characteristics of type a botulinum toxin in clinical use. *Botulinum J* 1 (1): 153–166.

7 Carruthers, J., Fagien, S., Matarasso, S.L. et al. (2004). Consensus recommendations on the use of botulinum toxin type a in facial aesthetics. *Plast Reconstr Surg* 114 (suppl 6): 1S–22S.

8 Goodman, G. (1998). Botulinum toxin for the correction of hyperkinetic facial lines. *Australas J Dermatol* 39: 158–163.

9 Carruthers, A. and Carruthers, J. (1998). Clinical indications and injection technique for the cosmetic use of botulinum a exotoxin. *Dermatol Surg* 24: 1189–1194.

10 Xeomin(incobotulinumtoxinA) [prescribing information]. Frankfurt am Main: Merz Pharmaceuticals, LLC; 2013.

11 Dysport®(abobotulinumtoxinA) [prescribing information]. Boulogne-Billancourt: Ipsen Biopharm Ltd; 2012.

12 Ipsen, Ltd. Dysport Summary of Product Characteristics [webpage on the Internet]. Surrey, UK: Datapharm Communications Ltd; 2013. Available from: www.medicines.org.uk/emc/medicine/870. Accessed July 13, 2013.

13 BOTOX® (onabotulinumtoxinA) [prescribing information]. Irvine, CA: Allergan, Inc.; 2013.

14 Hatheway, C. (1989). Bacterial sources of clostridial neurotoxins. In: *Botulinum Neurotoxin and Tetanus Toxin* (ed. L.L. Simpson), 4–24. San Diego, CA: Academic Press.

15 Inoue, K., Fujinaga, Y., Watanabe, T. et al. (1996). Molecular composition of Clostridium botulinum type a progenitor toxins. *Infect Immun* 64 (5): 1589–1594.

16 Eisele, K.H., Fink, K., Vey, M. et al. (2011). Studies on the dissociation of botulinum neurotoxin type a complexes. *Toxicon* 57 (4): 555–565.

17 Chen, F., Kuziemko, G.M., Amersdorfer, P. et al. (1997). Antibody mapping to domains of botulinum neurotoxin serotype a in the complexed and uncomplexed forms. *Infect Immun* 65 (5): 1626–1630.

18 Jiang, H.Y., Chen, S., Zhou, J. et al. (2014). Diffusion of two botulinum toxins type a on the forehead: double-blinded, randomized, controlled study. *Dermatol Surg* 40: 184–192.

19 Göschel, H., Wohlfarth, K., Frevert, J. et al. (1997). Botulinum a toxin therapy: neutralizing and nonneutralizing antibodies – therapeutic consequences. *Exp Neurol* 147 (1): 96–102.

20 Kukreja, R., Chang, T.W., Cai, S. et al. (2009). Immunological characterization of the subunits of type a botulinum neurotoxin and different components of its associated proteins. *Toxicon* 53 (6): 616–624.

21 Joshi, S.G., Elias, M., Singh, A. et al. (2011). Modulation of botulinum toxin-induced changes in neuromuscular function with antibodies directed against recombinant polypeptides or fragments. *Neuroscience* 179: 208–222.

22 Jiang, H.Y., Chen, S., Zhou, J. et al. (2014). Diffusion of two botulinum toxins type a on the forehead: double-blinded, randomized, controlled study. *Dermatol Surg* 40: 184–192.

23 McLellan, K., Das, R.E., Ekong, T.A. et al. (1996). Therapeutic botulinum type a toxin: factors affecting potency. *Toxicon* 34 (9): 975–985.

24 Cliff, S.H., Judodihardjo, H., and Eltringham, E. (2008). Different formulations of botulinum toxin type a have different migration characteristics: a double-blind, randomized study. *J Cosmet Dermatol* 7 (1): 50–54.

25 Pickett, A., Dodd, S., and Rzany, B. (2008). Confusion about diffusion and the art of misinterpreting data when comparing different botulinum toxins used in aesthetic applications. *J Cosmet Laser Ther* 10 (3): 181–183.

26 Carruthers, A., Carruthers, J., and Said, S. (2005). Dose-ranging study of botulinum toxin type A in the treatment of glabellar rhytids in females. *Dermatol Surg* 31 (4): 414–422. discussion 422. Biologics.

27 Ascher, B., Zakine, B., Kestemont, P. et al. (2004). A multicenter, randomized, double-blind, placebo-controlled study of efficacy and safety of 3 doses of botulinum toxin a in the treatment of glabellar lines. *J Am Acad Dermatol* 51 (2): 223–233.

28 Fulford-Smith, A., Gallagher, C.J., and Brin, M.F. (2013). Multicentre, randomized, phase III study of a single dose of incobotulinumtoxinA, free from complexing proteins, in the treatment of glabellar frown lines. *Derm Surg* 39 (7): 1118–1119.

29 Sampaio, C., Costa, J., and Ferreira, J.J. (2004). Clinical comparability of marketed formulations of botulinum toxin. *Mov Disord* 19 (Suppl 8): S129–S136.

30 Alam, M., Bolotin, D., Carruthers, J. et al. (2015). Consensus statement regarding storage and reuse of previously reconstituted neuromodulators. *Dermatol Surg* 41: 321–326.

31 Wieder, J.M. and Moy, R.L. (1998). Understanding botulinum toxin. Surgical anatomy of the frown, forehead, and periocular region. *Dermatol Surg* 24: 1172–1174.

32 Frankel, A.S. and Kamer, F.M. (1998). Chemical browlift. *Arch Otolaryngol Head Neck Surg* 124: 321–323.

33 Huilgol, S.C., Carruthers, A., and Carruthers, J.D. (1999). Raising eyebrows with botulinum toxin. *Dermatol Surg* 25: 373–376.

34 Huang, W., Rogachefsky, A.S., and Foster, J.A. (2000). Browlift with botulinum toxin. *Dermatol Surg* 26: 55–60.

35 Gordon, R.W. (2009). BOTOX cosmetic for lip and perioral enhancement. *Dent Today* 28: 94–97.

36 Semchyshyn, N. and Sengelmann, R.D. (2003). Botulinum toxin a treatment of perioral rhytides. *Dermatol Surg* 29: 490–495.

37 Carruthers, J. and Carruthers, A. (2003). Aesthetic botulinum a toxin in the mid and lower face and neck. *Dermatol Surg* 29: 468–476.

38 Beer, K., Yohn, M., and Closter, J. (2005). A double-blinded, placebo-controlled study of Botox for the treatment of subjects with chin rhytids. *J Drugs Dermatol* 4: 417–422.

39 Carruthers, J. and Carruthers, A. (2004). Botulinum toxin a in the mid and lower face and neck. *Dermatol Clin* 22: 151–158.

40 Hoefflin, S.M. (1998). Anatomy of the platysma and lip depressor muscles. A simplified mnemonic approach. *Dermatol Surg* 24: 1225–1231.

41 Matarasso, A. and Matarasso, S.L. (2003). Botulinum a exotoxin for the management of platysma bands. *Plast Reconstr Surg* 112 (suppl 5): 138S–140S.

42 Kane, M.A. (2003). Nonsurgical treatment of platysma bands with injection of botulinum toxin a revisited. *Plast Reconstr Surg* 112 (suppl 5): 125S–126S.

43 Batniji, R.K. and Falk, A.N. (2004). Update on botulinum toxin use in facial plastic and head and neck surgery. *Curr Opin Otolaryngol Head Neck Surg* 12: 317–322.

44 Hsu, T.S., Dover, J.S., Kaminer, M.S. et al. (2003). Why make patients exercise facial muscles for 4 hours after botulinum toxin treatment? *Arch Dermatol* 139: 948.

3

Cosmetic Fillers

Alexandra Radu and Faisal A. Quereshy

Oral and Maxillofacial Surgery, Case Western Reserve University, School of Dental Medicine, Cleveland, OH, USA

According to the American Society of Plastic Surgeons, there were 17.1 million cosmetic procedures performed in 2016, with 15.4 million of those qualifying as minimally invasive procedures. These numbers represent a 3% increase in minimally invasive procedures since 2015, and a 180% increase since 2000 [1]. More so, soft facial fillers made it to the top five minimally invasive procedures in 2016, with an increase of 2% since 2015, and an increase of 298% since 2000 [1]. Evidently, there is an escalating demand for cosmetic procedures that carry less risk, discomfort and need for down-time. Therefore, it is important for practitioners to have a detailed knowledge of facial fillers, their origin, indications, uses, and risks.

3.1 History of Cosmetic Fillers

The principles of facial augmentation have modified over the years as our understanding of the aging face has progressed. Whereas the early views saw aging as a superficial process mainly affected by gravity and the laxity of collagen, we understand now that aging happens at different levels in the structure of the face. The main culprit of aging face is the redistribution of fat throughout the face that transforms the smooth primary arcs and convexities of the young face in concavities, or flat planes that create the typical sharply demarcated hills and valleys of the aging face [2]. Therefore, rather than only focusing on the superficial rhytids and wrinkles caused by facial deformities, we have to understand that aging is a multifactorial process that involves environmental factors, dermal thinning, and even bone resorption.

The distribution of fat differs between the young and the aging face in that in the young face the superficial and deep fat are evenly distributed forming a homogenous appearance. The selective fat atrophy and hypertrophy of the aging face are responsible for the concavities and flat lines that create the characteristic flat lips, sunken temples and cheeks or scalloped mandible [2]. Fat atrophy first becomes visible in the temple areas and cheeks, and is then followed by chin and mandible. The excess skin follows the new face contours and, therefore, becomes sagging in the inferior and diagonal directions, from the temples towards the perioral region (Figure 3.1). In attempting to reestablish the contours of the young face, we must consider replenishing the atrophied fat of the face. The augmentation can be performed using a variety of cosmetic procedures and implantation

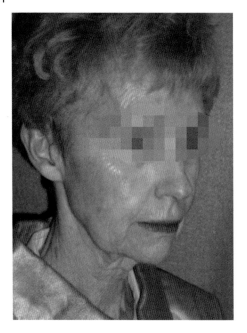

Figure 3.1 Patient illustrating fat atrophy creating hollow temples and cheeks, and skin laxity in the inferior and diagonal directions.

techniques. This section discusses cosmetic fillers for facial augmentation.

3.1.1 Emergence of Autologous Fillers

The use of soft tissue fillers dates from the late nineteenth century. The first physician to use soft tissue augmentation was Neuber in 1893 when he used a block of free fat harvested from the arms to reconstruct facial defects. His technique was modified later on by Lexer in 1910 when he started using single large block grafts to treat a malar depression and a receding chin. Lexer reported excellent short- and long-term results with very large fat grafts, but reported that approximately 66% of the graft resorbed and, therefore, significant overcorrection of the defect should be considered [3]. His encouraging results, however, could not be later reproduced by his colleagues. In 1911, Bruning used the same autologous fat for injection in the subcutaneous space, making him the first one to inject small amounts of fat in the subcutaneous space [4]. Later in the mid-1900s, an experiment using the free fat injections was analyzed to obtain 50% of the grafts viable at one year follow-up. At this time, many practitioners went away from using free fat grafts for augmentation of facial defects.

However, with the advent of liposuction techniques, free fat grafts once again became popular towards the end of the twentieth century when Fischer and Fischer described harvesting fat with the use of a "cellusuctiotome" to remove fat from riding breeches deformities [5]. The technique was further advanced by Yves-Gerard Illouz and his colleague Pierre Fournier throughout the 1980s, but it wasn't until Klein's introduction of tumescent anesthesia that the field of liposuction and fat transplantation took off [4]. This technique not only revolutionized liposuction surgery, but the field of facial augmentation by allowing the surgeon to obtain large volumes of free fat in a consistency that could be then injected in other parts of the body. Fournier added to Klein's technique by utilizing a micro cannula for obtaining the fat, but it wasn't until Asken that the harvested fat was used for the augmentation of facial defects [6]. Asken found that 90% of the fat extracted by liposuction appears viable as long as it is not traumatized either by improper handling or by the high suction pressure of the graft. It's the contribution of Klein, Fournier and Asken that have allowed the field of microlipoinjection to start expanding towards the1990s [4, 6].

3.1.2 Emergence of Non-autologous Fillers

The use of non-autologous grafts used for facial cosmetics has its beginnings at the end of nineteenth century with Gersuny who first injected a low-melting point paraffin in the scrotum of a young man to successfully form a testicular prosthesis [7]. He noted later that there was extensive migration and inflammatory reactions associated with the material. By the beginning of the twentieth century, it became obvious that paraffin was not going to be the preferred filler due to its high incidence of undesirable foreign body granuloma formation. Paraffin injections were therefore abandoned by 1920 in the Western world, but continued to be used in some Asian countries until the 1960s [4].

3.1.2.1 Silicones

Silicones were the next injectable product used for facial augmentation during the 1940s, with a tumultuous history following their introduction. The first injection of liquid silicone was performed in Japan. However, much of the silicones used early on were mixed with other substances, such as mineral oils or olive oil, resulting in many severe complications, such as foreign body and allergic reactions. The first injectable silicone in the US was introduced in 1960 by Dow Corning for repair of facial tissue augmentation [4]. The frequent presence of contaminants and the subsequent adverse reactions they caused, made the FDA withdraw liquid silicones from the American market towards the end of the 1990s [8]. Today, silicone fillers are compounds of long polymers of dimethylsiloxanes that are composed of methane, oxygen and elemental silica and they are approved for the correction of nasolabial folds, marionette lines, mid malar depression, and HIV lipoatrophy.

3.1.2.2 Bovine Collagen

In the 1970s, the research into collagen production led to the use of bovine collagen for the purpose of clinical augmentation, and implicitly, for facial augmentations [9]. The beginning of extracting bovine collagen started with Gross and Kirk who extracted collagen from fresh calf skin in 1958 [4]. They were able to produce a solid gel from the extracted collagen by gently warming the liquid collagen slowly to body temperature. The problem of antigenicity to bovine

collagen molecules was not solved until the 1960s when the removal of helical amino and carboxy terminal telopeptides from the collagen gel allowed it to be injected in humans [4]. In 1977, the first successful injection of collagen was performed by Knupp, Luck and Daniels. They reported that the collagen grafts remained stable and were progressively infiltrated by a matrix of viable host connective tissue. Later on, they injected the bovine collagen into the dermal and subcutaneous planes to correct depressed acne scars, subcutaneous atrophy, wrinkling and viral pock marks in 28 humans. The collagen fillers showed a 50–85% improvement that lasted for 3–18 months [10].

Zyderm I Collagen Implant (ZC-I) has been in use in the USA since 1977, even though it was not FDA approved until 1981. Zyderm must be place in the superficial dermal layer in a smooth even flow to achieve the desired correction. Klein's research led to the development of Zyplast that is placed in the mid-dermis for correction of deeper facial defect. Both Zyderm and Zyplast have remained the gold standards of injectable fillers and are standards against which newer materials are measured [4].

3.1.2.3 Porcine Collagen

Porcine collagen was only briefly used in the USA. It's resemblance to human collagen allowed for less risk for an allergic reaction and patients were not required to get skin testing prior to injection. Porcine collagen has been used outside USA since 2004. It gained popularity in the USA for about one year from 2008 to 2009. Currently, there are no available facial fillers on the American market based on porcine collagen [8].

3.1.2.4 Polymethylmethacrylate (PMMA)

PMMA is a synthetic material that is used in medicine and dentistry for bone cement, dentures and artificial eye lenses. When polymerized, the PMMA forms

30–40 µm spheres that can then be suspended in collagen for injection into facial defects. The collagen only serves as a delivery mechanism for the PMMA beads, and it degrades after injection into the soft tissue, leaving just the PMMA beads to become the permanent implant. The injectable compound is a suspension composed of 20% non-resorbable PMMA and 80% bovine collagen. The compound started being used in the 1980, but it wasn't until 1995 that a prospective study using 118 patients indicating a high patient satisfaction (90%) with results of treatment lasting a minimum of two years [11].

3.1.2.5 Hyaluronic Acid

Hyaluronic acid is a polysaccharide found naturally in the dermis of all mammals. The compound consists of regular repeating non-sulfate disaccharide units of glucuronic acid and N-acetylglucosamine that has the ability to bond water and it can help assist the skin to improve its hydration and increase turgor. Hyaluronic acid is a compound identical across mammalian species and is produced in many different types of cells [4]. The fact that hyaluronic acid exhibits no tissue or species specificity is crucial to minimize any immunologic reactions or transplantation rejection. While collagen fillers remained very popular in the 1980s and 1990s, European practitioners were starting to use hyaluronic acid fillers more and more. In a multicenter clinical study initiated in 1991, Piacquadio reported the use of cross-linked hyaluronic acid in 150 patients to augment facial deformities such as wrinkles or scars. The study found 84% moderate improvement, and 80% patient satisfaction at 12-week follow-up [12]. Hylaform is the first FDA approved hyaluronic acid facial filler and it became available on the American market in 2004. Since the emergence of this product on the market, hyaluronic acid fillers have grown in popularity and are currently some of the most commonly used facial fillers in the United States, with numerous brands used for different facial deficiencies.

3.1.2.6 Dextran Beads in Hyaluronic Acid

In this facial filler, dextran microspheres form micro particles with a positively charged surface and a diameter of approximately 80–120 µm that are suspended in hyaluronic acid. The hyaluronic acid in this compound is biodegradable and it acts as a delivery system to support the relatively large dextran molecules [13]. The compound was first introduced in Europe in 2004, and it has never been FDA approved for use in the USA.

3.1.2.7 Poly-L-lactic Acid

Poly-L-lactic acid is a biodegradable, synthetic polymer of L-lactic acid, which has been used in the medical field for over 40 years. The compound was first used in different medical devices, such as reabsorbable plates, screws, and suture materials. The filler consists of poly-L-lactic acid microspheres that stimulate the formation of type I collagen, mannitol, and sodium carboxymethylcellulose, completed with sterile water for injection [9]. Unlike other dermal fillers that are intended to correct discrete facial wrinkles or folds, poly-L-lactic acid provides volumetric expansion of volume-deficient areas [9]. This product has been FDA approved in the USA since 2004 as a soft tissue filler for lipoatrophy of cheeks, and for HIV patients who are under highly active antiviral therapy.

3.1.2.8 Calcium Hydroxylapatite

Calcium hydroxylapatite is composed of a suspension of 30% synthetic calcium hydroxylapatite microspheres of 25–45 µm diameter, suspended in a 70% gel consisting of 36.6% sterile water, 1.3% sodium carboxymethyl cellulose and 6.4% glycerin [14]. This product has been used in medicine for over 20 years, and it is currently FDA approved for use in oral maxillofacial defects, and laryngeal and vocal fold augmentation. However, the use as a facial filler is only an off-label function of the calcium hydroxylapatite.

3.1.2.9 Polyvinyl Microspheres Suspended in Polyacrylamide

This compound is a suspension of 6% polyvinyl hydroxide microspheres suspended in 2.5% polyacrylamide hydrogel. This facial filler is available in Europe only, and it has not been FDA-approved for use in the USA for facial augmentation [9].

3.1.2.10 Polytetrafluoroethylene (PTFE)

Polytetrafluoroethylene (Teflon) paste is a facial filler used for facial augmentation and rhinoplasty augmentation. Robert W. Gore and William L. Gore developed expanded polytetrafluoroethylene (e-PTFE) as an expanded fibrillated form of polytetrafluoroethylene. Expanded polytetrafluoroethylene was FDA approved in 1991 [15] and used for nasolabial fold and rhytid correction.

3.1.2.11 Polyoxyethylene and Polyoxypropylene

This facial filler is a block co-polymer of polyoxyethylene and polyoxypropylene with mineral salts, amino acids, and vitamins. The compound is a liquid that becomes a gel upon injection in the soft tissue. This compound has been used in Europe for facial augmentation but it is not FDA approved as a facial filler in the USA.

3.2 Classification

With the increased demand in soft tissue fillers, a myriad of companies have developed and manufactured products throughout the world. The Food and Drug Administration regulates the use of facial fillers in the USA, but there are fillers that are being used off-label for facial augmentation. Many facial fillers have similar indications and properties, and the preference for using one product over another can come from patients or practitioners alike.

Cosmetic soft tissue fillers can be broadly classified based on the origin of the graft (autologous vs. nonautologous), the mechanism of metabolism (biodegradable vs. nonbiodegradable), longevity (permanent vs. semi-permanent) or components (organic vs. synthetic). Each of these classifications benefit further from subdivisions to be able to include the different products available on the market today.

3.2.1 Biodegradable Facial Fillers

Biodegradable soft tissue fillers are capable of being metabolized by human enzymes and are absorbed following cutaneous injection (Table 3.1). The clinical effects are typically short lived and they generally do not create granulomatous reactions. These materials are derived from synthetic or natural means and some may be used as a trigger mechanism to boost fibroblast and collagen production [14].

3.2.2 Autologous and Allogeneic Facial Fillers

The most frequently discussed autologous facial filler is the free fat graft. However, there are commercial products that are also classified as autologous facial fillers. One such product is Autologen, which is a true autologous dermal implant that is aseptically prepared from the patient's own tissue of intact collagen fibrils, elastic tissue and proteoglycans. Autologen is manufactured from the patient's own skin. One cc of Autologen is fabricated from three square inches of skin. Isolagen and Plasmagel are two similar products that are created from the patient's fibroblasts and blood plasma, respectively.

Allorderm is an acellular freeze-dried human cadaver dermis processed from donors who have been previously screened and inactivated for viral infections. The

Table 3.1 Most popular classes of biodegradable cosmetic fillers on the market, together with the marketable brand names and the most commonly cited indications.

Composition	Common commercial brands	General indications	FDA approval
Fat	Autologous fat and dermis-fat grafting	Correction of nasolabial folds, cheeks, and marionette lines	Not applicable
Human collagen	CosmoDerm I,II Isolagen Cymetra and Alloderm Fascian	Injection into the superficial papillary dermis for correction of soft tissue contour deficiencies, such as wrinkles and acne scars	CosmoDerm – 2003
Porcine collagen	Fibroquel Permacol Evolence	Correction of moderate to deep facial wrinkles, and folds, such as the nasolabial folds	Evolence – 2008
Bovine collagen	Zyderm I&II, Zyplast Koken Atelocollagen Endoplast 50	Depressed scars, facial contour enhancement (including lips), dermal atrophy from disease or corticosteroid injections, wrinkles, creases, lines caused by facial expression or aging Used in mid to deep dermal tissues for correction of contour deficiencies	Zyderm - 1981 Zyplast – 1985
Hyaluronic acid	Hylaform, Hylaform Plus, Hylaform Fineline Juvederm 18,24,30 Captique Rofilan Hylan Gel AcHyal Matridur Hyal-System Puragen	Injection into the mid to deep dermis for correction of moderate to severe facial wrinkles and folds (such as nasolabial folds). Moderate to severe facial lines, folds and wrinkles	Juvederm – 2010/2013/2016/2017 Restylane – 2011/2014/2015 Belotero – 2011 Prevelle – 2008 Eeless – 2006 Captique – 2004 Hylaform – 2004
Dextran beads in hyaluronic acid	Matridex Reviderm intra	Correction of facial wrinkles and folds (glabella folds, lip contour, lip augmentation, oral commissures, fine line, perioral lines, nasolabial folds) and contour correction Correction of smoker lines, premolar lines above the top lip and laughter lines around the eyes	Pending FDA approval
Poly-L-lactic acid	New-fill Sculptra	Off-label used for temples, upper zygoma, nasolabial and malar regions, periorbital and preauricular regions, and for the jaw line.	Sculptra – 2004/2009
Calcium Hydroxylapatite	Radiesse	Soft tissue filling of the nasolabial folds, facial lipodystrophy, wrinkles, globular lines, scars and liposuction contour defects	Radiesse – 2006/2015

material is obtained from the American Association of Tissue Banks and it was initially used to treat burn victims in need of full-thickness dermal transplantations [4].

3.2.3 Xenograft Facial Fillers

While fat is the oldest facial filler, bovine collagen (Zyderm I, Zyderm II and Zyplast) have been the most used prepackaged injectable fillers. Xenograft collagen fillers, however, are not currently used anymore, and they have been replaced by other fillers. One of the main reason for discontinuing bovine collagen filler is the high risk for allergic reactions. A double skin test spread four weeks apart was needed prior to injection of the bovine based collagen filler. Since porcine collagen is closer related to human collagen, no allergy testing was needed. However, porcine collagen fillers were also removed from the market to make space for other superior compounds.

Injectable hyaluronic acid gel is a viscous clear material that can be derived from avian tissue or by fermentation of *Streptococci* bacteria [9]. It is one of the most versatile facial fillers on the market today, and comes in different formulations with many varied indications, used for small or large volume defects. Hyaluronic acid can also be used as a suspension for dextran beads. This facial filler, however, is more popular in non-US markets and has never received FDA approval.

3.2.4 Synthetic Facial Fillers

The two most commonly used facial fillers in this category are poly-L-lactic acid and calcium hydroxylapatite. Poly-L-lactic acid is an injectable resorbable polymer that stimulates a fibrous tissue response that in turn produces volume increase in deficient areas of the face. Therefore, poly-L-lactic acid does not provide mechanical correction of volume defects, but instead induces a host reaction that corrects the deficiencies. Hydroxylapatite fillers act similarly to hyaluronic acid fillers, but with greater viscosity, therefore, being used to correct larger volume deficiencies.

3.2.5 Nonbiodegradable Facial Fillers

Nonbiodegradable facial fillers represent a group of products that cannot be metabolized by human enzymes and, therefore, persist indefinitely in tissue. While longevity is traditionally a main advantage of this group, they generally create more severe cutaneous adverse reactions, as it will be detailed later in the chapter.

Paraffin is a compound that is usually mentioned only for its contribution in the development of synthetic, nonbiodegradable facial fillers. However, very early on it was decided that the benefits of this filler do not overcome its potential side effects, such as the high occurrence of connective tissue disease due to the foreign tissue reactions. Similarly, silicone (Silikon 1000, SilSkin 1000) is not a favorite in this category because the impurities often found in injectable silicones have the high risk of creating the same adverse foreign tissue reactions.

Artecol is a mixture of biodegradable (bovine collagen) and non-biodegradable components (PMMA spheres). However, it is usually classified as a synthetic compound that is not resorbed by the body. As discussed previously, the delivery mechanism, the bovine collagen is resorbed by the soft tissue.

Polytetrafluoroethylene (PTFE) and expanded polytetrafluoroethylene (e-PTFE) are products that are not commonly used in the USA for facial augmentation. They have, however, a long history in cardiac and vascular surgery (Table 3.2).

3.3 Ease of Use

The ideal facial filler should not only provide good esthetic results, but it should also be manageable for practitioners in order to obtain predictable results with

Table 3.2 Most popular classes of nonbiodegradable cosmetic fillers on the market, together with the marketable brand names and the most commonly cited indications.

Composition	Common commercial brands	General indications	FDA approval
Saturated hydrocarbons	Paraffin	Augmentation of large volume deficiencies	No FDA approval Not in use
Silicon	MDX-4-4011 Dow Corning PMS 350 Silikon 1000 SilSkin 1000	Correction of the nasolabial folds, marionette lines, mid-molar depression and HIV lipoatrophy	No FDA approval for facial augmentation Off-label use
PMMA	Bioplastique Arteplast Artecoll Artefill Aphrodite gold	Correction of facial rhytids, subdermal defects and chin augmentation	Artefill – 2006
Polyvinil microspheres suspended in polyacrylamide	Metacril DermaLive and DermaDeep Aquamid Interfall Bio-Alcamid	Lip augmentation	No FDA approval
PTFE/e-PTFE	Teflon Advanta GORE S.A.M. SoftForm and UltraFost	Augmentation of lips and nasolabial folds, correction of rhytids	Gore S.A.M. – 1991
Polyoxyethylene and polyoxypropylene	Profil	Soft tissue augmentation	No FDA approval

every use. Preferably, the product should come in prepackaged syringes, it should not require special storage and it should not require dilution prior to injection.

The use of free fat grafts for cosmetic facial augmentation has gone through several developmental stages over the years. Fat could be removed with a syringe or aspirator, not employing tumescent anesthesia, and simply returned to the host. With the introduction of tumescent anesthesia, however, surgeons can take advantage of micro cannulas (2–3 mm in diameter) with nonabrasive tips that allow harvesting of free fat with minimal trauma to the surrounding structures. The fat could then be returned to the host without risks of rejection or formation of foreign body reactions. The harvesting

procedure does not add significant morbidity to the donor site due to the modern instrumentation and the use of tumescent anesthesia. Syringe aspiration with a handheld 10 ml or larger syringe can also be used. The plunger has to be held 2–3 ml for a low vacuum pressure that allows atraumatic removal. After harvesting, the aspirate is positioned upright for 15 minutes or more to allow separation into a supernatant and infranatant fraction. The infranatant fluid is then drained off. The areas that can benefit most from autologous fat grafts are the nasolabial folds, cheeks, and marionette lines. Autologen, Isolgaen and Plasmagel are superficially placed products and are, therefore, applicable for fine lines, wrinkles, depressions, and lip augmentation.

Bovine collagen based fillers are easy to inject and can provide excellent results for depressed acne scars, nasolabial folds, and lips. PMMA and bovine collagen suspension is also FDA approved for the correction of nasolabial folds. It has, however, other off-label uses for correction of deep facial wrinkles at other sites of the face. Since injectable PMMA contains 0.3% lidocaine, there is no need for additional local anesthesia. The PMMA is supplied in 0.8 or 0.4 ml syringes, and it is recommended that a 26-gauge needle is used for injection. PMMA is injected into the dermal-subcutaneous junction utilizing the "tunneling" or "linear threading technique." After injection, the area should be massaged to eliminate any accumulations of the suspension that may be felt subcutaneously. Optimal corrections with PMMA often requires multiple treatments.

Hyaluronic acid fillers represent a recent breakthrough for augmentation, not requiring allergy testing, and providing a longer duration than most previous collagen fillers. Hyaluronic injectables come in prepackaged syringes that do not require further manipulation. It is recommended to use a smaller needle (30–32 gauge) for more superficial placement of the fillers, and a larger needle (27 gauge) for placement of more viscous filler in the deeper layers needing volume correction. This filler can be combined with other cosmetic products and may be layered with other hyaluronic facial fillers, or with other cosmetic fillers.

Poly-L-lactic acid is injected into the deep dermis or subcutaneous layer using a 26-gauge needle with a tunneling technique, and massage of the product is recommended after injection. No overcorrection is usually required when using poly-L-lactic acid fillers, but most patients will need several series of injections spaced one to two months apart [14]. One vial is diluted with water, and may be mixed with lidocaine to eliminate the need for topical anesthesia or nerve blocks prior to injection of the filler. Additionally, lidocaine reduces edema and ecchymosis by inhibiting the activation of eosinophils.

Calcium hydroxylapatite is a sterile, latex-free, non-pyrogenic, semi-solid, cohesive subdermal, injectable implant that is supplied in 1.3 ml disposal syringes. After injection into the facial defects, the gel is dissipated and replaced with soft tissue growth, while the calcium hydroxylapatite remains at the site of injection [16]. When injected as small microspheres, calcium hydroxylapatite acts as a scaffold that promotes new tissue formation similar to its surrounding environment. Local anesthetic with 1% Lidocaine with 1 : 100 000 epinephrine along the site of the injection can provide patient comfort prior to injection of the filler.

Polyvinyl microspheres suspended in polyacrylamide is a filler mostly used for lip augmentation and it is injected in the dermis or subcutis [16]. It flows uniformly in the deficient space and is generally considered easy to use.

3.4 Benefits

In order for a compound to be considered adequate for augmentation of facial defects, it must meet certain criteria. First, the compound must be considered safe for patients. Therefore, it must be nonteratogenic, noncarcinogenic and it must not cause severe adverse local and systemic reactions. Furthermore, the agent must provide predictable, persistent correction through reproducible implantation techniques, with no migration of the substance in the soft tissue. Also, the ideal filler should be painless on injection, and be free from all transmissible diseases [17]. The FDA regulates these products and assures users that the composition of the fillers is pure and harmless for use in facial augmentation. However, not one filler possesses all the benefits of the ideal fillers. They all have individual benefits and it's important to recognize them in order to make the right choice.

The main benefit of fat grafts used for facial augmentation is that they carry virtually no risk for allergic reactions or rejection. Unlike the animal-derived collagen fillers and synthetic fillers, the fat transferred to the face belongs to the patient and therefore the body will not perceive it as a foreign object. Another benefit associated with autologous fat transfers is the long-lasting effects. Even though the rate of resorption is variable among patients, the fat that remains grafted in the subcutaneous tissue can last for several years after the procedure, without the need for frequent revision (Figure 3.2). Similarly, Autologen,

(a)   (b)

(c)   (d)

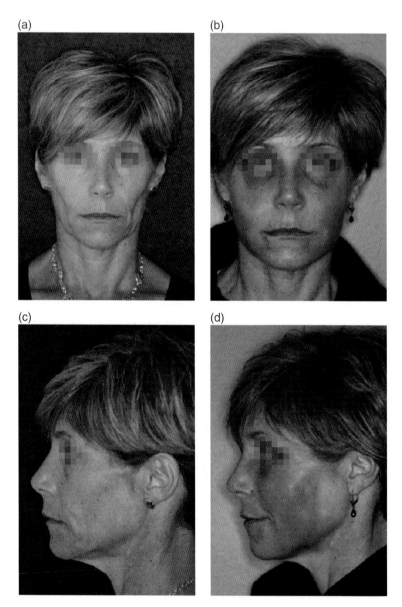

Figure 3.2 Facial augmentation using free fat graft. (a,c) Patient before treatment in frontal and profile positions. (b,d) Patient after injection of autologous fat in the malar, perioral, and infraorbital regions (Post-operative day 4).

Isolagen, and Plasmagel have greater longevity than bovine collagen because of the impact of autologous composition. Free fat grafts can also be combined with other facial rejuvenation products, such as Botox. Augmentation using the patient's own fat harvest also provides a cost benefit since the patient does not have to pay for the products purchased from the pharmaceutical companies.

One of the biggest benefits of using PMMA based fillers is the longevity of the suspension. The correction of nasolabial folds has been reported to last within a range of 5–10 years. Also, due to its easy technique and inert character, this is an easy product to use.

Hyaluronic acid fillers are a popular choice for facial augmentation mainly for the low risk for allergic reactions, ease of use, and treatment longevity. The results are seen immediately after injecting the filler in the facial defects (Figure 3.3). Also, the availability of hyaluronic acid in multiple viscosities allow for the practitioners to achieve new levels of facial esthetics. The high viscosity low molecular weight hyaluronic acid has advantages when used for volume restorations (Figure 3.4),

including versatility of use (differential facial planes), high malleability, minimal swelling, limited downtime, and immediate patient satisfaction [17]. Based on the type of hyaluronic acid, the longevity of the treatment can vary from 3 to 12 months with the higher molecular weight hyaluronic acid having the greater longevity. The adding of the cross-linked dextran to the hyaluronic mix increases the longevity of the facial filler to up to two years [13].

The main advantage for using poly-L-lactic acid is the low risk for allergic reactions due to the fact that the product is not animal based. Therefore, no allergy testing is necessary before the injection of the compound. More so, poly-L-lactic acid is a medium-term filer, lasting between 18 and 24 months after a series of injections [18].

Calcium hydroxylapatite is a biodegradable substance, and is metabolized by the body in a similar fashion as bone. Therefore, it has an excellent tolerance and it creates minimal, if any, inflammatory response with no foreign body reaction and without evidence of local or systemic toxicity. After 12–18 months post-injection the achieved volumes begin

(a)

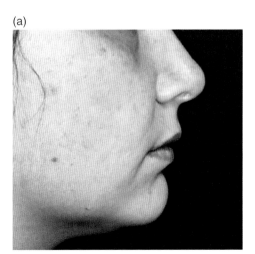

(b)

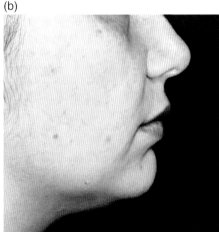

Figure 3.3 Volume lip augmentation using hyaluronic acid. (a) Patient before treatment. (b) Three days post-operatively after initial edema has resolved.

(a) (b)

(c) (d)

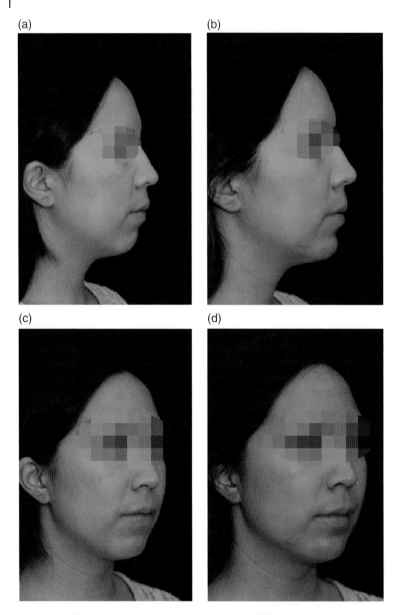

Figure 3.4 Chin augmentation using hyaluronic acid filler. (a,c) Patient before treatment in frontal and three quarters positions. (b,d) Patient immediately after injection of hyaluronic acid in the chin.

to diminish, through some results can be noted 24 months post injection. The average longevity reported for this facial filler is 12–18 months. There is high patient satisfaction with this product, with 87% of patients reporting very good results in preliminary studies [16].

3.5 Complications

The complications associated with the use of soft tissue fillers can be classified as immediate and delayed. Immediate complications occur within days of the procedure, whereas delayed complications can appear

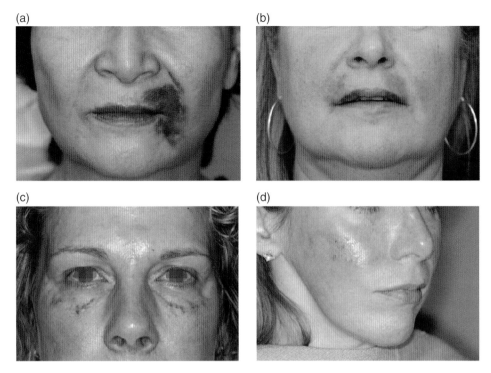

Figure 3.5 Complications following injection of facial fillers. (a,b) Ecchymosis following lip augmentation. (c) Injection marks evident immediately after injection in the periorbital region. (d) Cheek edema after hyaluronic acid augmentation.

from weeks to years after the procedure. Common adverse reactions for all facial fillers are related to the injection of the fillers, such as pain, bruising, bleeding, erythema after injection, and treatment asymmetries (Figure 3.5). Lumpiness and dimpling are usually associated with superficial injection of fillers and are usually resolvable by massaging the area of concern [9]. Other rare complications associated with the use of fillers are infection, hematoma formation, granuloma formation, nodules, migration, or extrusion. Granulomas are usually treated with injection of steroids, and sometimes may require surgical excision.

Biodegradable soft tissue fillers produce immediate and short-term cutaneous adverse reactions, such as infections, type I hypersensitivity reactions, and rarely granulomas. Because non-biodegradable soft tissue fillers stay longer at the site of injection, more long-term cutaneous

adverse reactions, such as granulomatous reactions may be seen more frequently. More so, because of their permanent nature and difficulty of removing the material, injectable synthetic polymers can produce significant complications that could become challenging to treat [19]. There are many overlapping complications among the different classes and brands of facial fillers, hence, a through discussion with the patient prior to the procedure is critical.

The main complication associated with the use of free fat grafts is the variable longevity of the grafts. It is supported by clinical experience that fat grafting is most successful when the graft is transferred in a region already occupied by adipose tissue [4]. The literature fails to provide definitive evidence of fat survival [23] with authors reporting fat survival in the 0–90% range [24]. Therefore, most practitioners currently prefer the use of fillers that have more predictable results in the long term. Finally, there have been reports where free fat filler injections into the glabellar region or nasolabial fold can cause retinal artery occlusion more so than other facial fillers [20].

The main complication related to bovine collagen fillers is the potential allergic reactions, requiring a double skin test prior to injection. Depending on the site of injection, collagen can last from two to six months. The duration of bovine collagen is longer in areas with decreased mobility, and it lowers in areas with increased mobility such as the lips.

Similarly to bovine collagen, the PMMA suspended in bovine collagen has a potential for allergic reactions. Therefore, patients have to undergo the same process of testing the bovine collagen six weeks, and then two weeks, prior to injection of the filler. The most common complications associated with PMMA are lumpiness, increased skin sensitivity, persistent edema or erythema and formation of granulomas. Because of the longevity of the PMMA fillers, the implantation of the suspension is less forgiving and the fillers must be placed with great care [9]. Due to its consistency, PMMA may be easily felt through the skin in patients with extremely thing and loose skin. Finally, injecting the filler into dermal vessels may cause vascular occlusion, infarction, or embolic phenomena.

Theoretically, the risk of an immune-mediated reaction is minimal when using hyaluronic acid fillers. However, there have been reports of immediate and delayed side effects to these compounds that have been recorded in the range of one week to one year after the procedure. Besides the transient non-allergic, local side effects that are generalized to all facial fillers (edema, ecchymosis, hypercorrection and bluish discoloration) other complications can be more serious and long term. For example, hyaluronic acid fillers

have been associated with tender granulomas and indurated nodules suggesting an allergic mechanism. However, in most recent years most of the attention has been given to biofilms, an infectious complication due to microorganisms with excretion of an extracellular protective adhesive matrix allowing development of antibiotic resistant microorganisms [25]. The dextran beads that can be added to the hyaluronic acid suspension have themselves the risk of inducing delayed inflammatory reactions at the local site of injection, and granuloma formation due to the foreign body reaction to the dextran beads [13].

The silicones have the potential of developing a diffuse epithelioid granulomatous infiltrate. This reaction pattern is described as "Swiss-cheese" like in appearance and may mimic liposarcoma. Moreover, the presence of impurities can create foreign body giant cells. The granulomatous reactions may also be seen at a distant site from the injected lesions site, because of migration of the soft tissue filler, and granulomas may be seen up to 16 years after injection [21].

No severe allergic reactions have been reported with using polyvinyl microspheres suspended in polyacrylamide. The polyvinyl microspheres form uniform cystic spaces around them [22]. However, the polyacrylamide is reabsorbed in approximately six months after injection.

There are several adverse reactions associated with the use of PTFE and e-PTFE. Foreign-body reactions have been reported with the use of PTFE paste with refractive filamentous foreign materials consistent with Teflon paste and a surrounding inflammatory infiltrate, or lymphocytes multinucleate giant cells. Similarly, granulomatous reactions have been reported with the use of e-PTFE, and on histology evaluation, e-PTFE threads are seen as filamentous and birefringent under polarizing microscope [26]. More so, there have been reports of fistula formation, extrusion of the implant

(Figure 3.6), infections, induration/granuloma formation and migration of the implant when using e-PTFE [16].

Calcium hydroxylapatite is considered a safe filler without any significant complications besides the unspecific complications noted with other fillers, such as transient lumpiness and localized edema/erythema.

Polyoxyethylene- and polyoxypropylene-based facial fillers have not been extensively studied in literature, but a common side effect reported by practitioners is lipoatrophy at the site of injection [16].

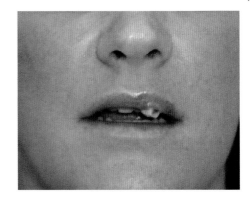

Figure 3.6 Extrusion of e-PTFE paste after lip augmentation.

References

1 American Society of Plastic Surgeons. 2016. Cosmetic & reconstructive procedure trends. Plastic Surgery Statistics. Retrieved on March 22, 2017 from https://d2wirczt3b6wjm.cloudfront.net/News/Statistics/2016/2016-plastic-surgery-statistics-report.pdf.

2 Burgess, C.M. (2006). Principles of soft tissue augmentation for the aging face. *Clinical Interventions in Aging* 1 (4): 349–355.

3 Lexer, E. (1919). Fatty tissue transplantation. In: *Die freien transplantation*, vol. 1 (ed. E. Lexer), 265–302. Stuttgart: Ferdinand Enke.

4 Klein, A.W. and Elson, M.L. (2000). The history of substances for soft tissue augmentation. *Dermatologic Surgery* 26 (12): 1096–1105.

5 Fischer, A. and Fischer, G.M. (1977). Revised technique for cellulitis fat. Reduction in riding breeches deformity. *Bulletin of the International Academy of Cosmetic Surgery* 2: 40–42.

6 Asken, S. (1987). Autologous fat transplantation: micro and macro techniques. *American Journal of Cosmetic Surgery* 4: 111–121.

7 Connell, G.F. (1903). The subcutaneous injection of paraffin for the correction of the deformities of the nose. *The Journal of the American Medical Association* 61 (12): 697–703.

8 Kotnis, T.C. and Rivnik, A. (2009). The history of injectable fillers. *Facial Plastic Surgery* 25 (2): 067–072.

9 Alam, M., Gladstone, H., Kramer, E.M. et al. (2008). ASDS guidelines of care: injectable fillers. *Dermatologic Surgery* 34 (1): 115–148.

10 Knapp, T.R., Kaplan, E.N., and Daniels, J.R. (1997). Injectable collagen for soft tissue augmentation. *Plastic Reconstructive Surgery* 60: 389.

11 Lamperle, G., Hazan-Gauthier, N., and Lamperle, M. (1995). PMMA microspheres (Artecoll) for skin and soft tissue augmentation. Part II. Clinical investigations. *Plastic and Reconstructive Surgery* 96: 627–634.

12 Picquadio, D. (1994). Crosslinked hyaluronic acid (hylan gel) as a soft tissue augmentation material: a preliminary assessment. In: *Evaluation and Treatment of the Aging Face*, 304–308. New York: Springer-Verlag.

13 Huh, S.Y., Cho, S., Kim, K.H. et al. (2010). A case of complication after Matridex injection. *Annals of Dermatology* 22 (1): 81–84.

14 Pfulg, M.E. and Le-Huu, S. (2010). Esthetic skin treatments (fillers). In: *Pastic and Reconstructive Surgery* (ed. M.Z. Siemionow and M. Eisenmann-Klein), 221–232. London: Springer-Verlag.

15 Sherris, D.A. and Larrabee, W.F. (1996). Expanded polytetrafluoroethylene augmentation of the lower face. *The Laryngoscope* 106 (5 Pt 1): 658–663.

16 Dadzie, O.E., Mahalingam, M., Parada, M. et al. (2007). *Journal of Cutaneous Pathology* 35: 536–548.

17 Muhn, C., Rosen, N., Solish, N. et al. (2012). The evolving role of hyaluronic acid fillers for facial volume restoration and contouring: a Canadian overview. *Clinical, Cosmetic and Investigational Dermatology* 5: 147–158.

18 Vleggaar, D. and Bauer, U. (2004). Facial enhancement and the European experience with Sculptra (poly-l-lactic acid). *Journal of Drugs in Dermatology* 3 (5): 542–547.

19 Maas, C.S., Papel, I.D., Greene, D. et al. (1997). Complications of injectable synthetic polymers in facial augmentation. *Dermatologic Surgery* 23 (10): 871–877.

20 Park, S.W., Woo, S.E., Park, K.H. et al. (2012). Iatrogenic retinal artery occlusion caused by cosmetic facial filler injections. *American Journal of Ophthalmology* 154 (4): 653–662.

21 Poveda, R., Began, J.V., Murillo, J. et al. (2004). Granulomatous facial reaction to injected cosmetic fillers – a presentation of five cases. *Oral Medicine, Oral Pathology and Oral Surgery* 11: E1–E5.

22 Wortsman, X. (2015). Identification and complications of cosmetic fillers. *Journal of Ultrasound in Medicine* 34 (7): 1163–1172.

23 Kauffman, M.R., Miller, T., Haung, C. et al. (2007). Autologous fat transfer for facial recontouring: is there science behind the art? *Plastic and Reconstructive Surgery* 119 (7): 2287–2296.

24 Samdal, F., Skolleborg, K.C., and Berthelsen, N. (1992). The effest of preoperative needle abrasion of the recipient on survival of autologous free fat grafts in rats. *Scandinavian Journal of Plastic and Reconstructive Surgery and Hand Surgery* 26 (1): 33–36.

25 Bitterman-Deutsch, O., Kogan, L., and Nasser, F. (2015). Delayed immune mediated adverse effects to hyaluronic acid fillers: reports of five cases and review of the literature. *Dermatology Reports* 7 (1): 51–58.

26 Lombardi, T., Samson, J., Plantier, F. et al. (2004). Orofacial granulomas after injection of cosmetic fillers. Histopathologic and clinical study of 11 cases. *Journal of Oral Pathology and Medicine* 33 (2): 115–120.

4

Hyaluronic Acid Dermal Fillers

Tirbod Fattahi and Salam Salman

Department of Oral and Maxillofacial Surgery, University of Florida, Jacksonville, FL, USA

4.1 Introduction

History of hyaluronic acid (HA) dermal fillers goes back to the late 1970s when the science of injectable skin fillers really began. Although the first HA filler was not formally introduced in the USA until the early 2000s, bovine collagen became the first injectable filler material in 1977 when Zyderm and Zyplast (Inamed Aesthetics, Santa Barbara, California) were introduced. Both derived from cow collagen, Zyderm and Zyplast became quite popular simply due to absence of any other competitor and their effectiveness in eliminating moderate to deep rhytids and augmenting soft tissue defects. Similar to today's HA fillers where scientific modification (crosslinking) of HA particles produces different products within the same family (Juvéderm Ultra vs. Juvéderm Ultra Plus), Zyplast was formulated to be the more "viscous" formulation, indicated for a deeper level of augmentation. The biggest drawback of bovine collagen injectables became the need for allergy testing. Although further enhancements of bovine collagen were performed (Zyplast 2), bovine collagen injectables eventually lost their luster and are no longer on the market. However, many manufacturers, both national and international, continued to look for safer and newer options for injectable dermal fillers. Finally, in 2003, Restylane (Galderma Laboratories, Fort Worth, Texas) became the first injectable HA filler approved in the USA. Since then, there have been over a dozen other HA dermal fillers that have entered the cosmetic surgery market with various degrees of success.

4.2 Hyaluronic Acid

The term HA is derived from *hyalos* (Greek for vitreous) and uronic acid since it is abundantly found in the vitreous fluid of the eye with a high concentration of uronic acid. HA, is a naturally occurring protein (glycosaminoglycan) component of the extracellular matrix throughout the human body. The HA peptide is a combination of repeating sequences of N-acetyl-glucosamine and glucuronic acid. The highest concentration (over 50%) is found in human skin, eyes, as well as joint spaces. It is estimated that a 70-kg male adult has about 15 g of HA in his body [1]. Because it is a hydrophilic protein, HA attracts water and maintains hydration wherever it is injected or naturally resides; this

Neurotoxins and Fillers in Facial Esthetic Surgery, First Edition. Edited by Bradford M. Towne and Pushkar Mehra.
Companion website: www.wiley.com/go/towne/neurotoxins

characteristic has high clinical value which will be discussed later. All HA particles also have rheologic properties (elasticity and viscosity) which is the critical advantage in management of oste-oarthritis, one of the earliest indication for HA injectable therapy.

The main type of HA used in cosmetic surgery today is known as *Non-Animal Stabilized Hyaluronic Acid* (NASHA). This formulation, as the name implies, does not have any animal products unlike some earlier HA injectables used in the treatment of retinal issues or arthritic conditions. This type of HA filler is typi-cally formulated in a gel-like consistency. The viscosity of this gel-like substance is directly influenced by cross-linking, the process of attaching multiple chains of HA together. Cross-linking will increase the particle size of HA fillers, which will increase their longevity and will make the fillers more viscous. More cross-linked fillers are more appropriate for deeper plane injections.

4.3   Available Products

The most commonly used HA fillers in the USA are the following:

- *Juvéderm* (Allergan, Irvine, California)
- *Perlane* (Galderma, Fort Worth, Texas)
- *Restylane* (Galderma, Fort Worth, Texas)
- *Belotero* (Merz, Raleigh, North Carolina)

Many of the manufacturers have created multiple types of fillers within the same family by modifying the cross-linking and/or particle size; this modification allows for various types of clinical indi-cations. For example, Juvéderm fillers are formulated as *Ultra*, *Ultra Plus*, or *Voluma*, all depending on the degree of cross-linking and particle size. Similarly, Restylane has been formulated as *Restylane*, *Restylane Silk*, and *Restylane Lyft*, again depending on particle size,

cross-linking, and clinical indications. Local anesthetic has also been added to the formulation of many HA fillers for pain control during the injection process. For example, Juvéderm Ultra *XC* contains xylocaine®.

4.4   Clinical Indications

HA dermal fillers are indicated for volume replacement and/or augmentation at the recipient site. As with most cosmetic injectables, including neurotoxins, most indications are not Food and Drug Administration (FDA) approved and are considered off-label use. It is up to the imagination of the clinician, the character-istics of the specific filler, and the location of the defect that determine the specific type of HA to use. Most common indica-tions for HA fillers in the face include:

- Nasolabial fold augmentation;
- Lip and lip-liner augmentation;
- Perioral rhytid augmentation;
- Tear trough augmentation;
- Cheek augmentation;
- Glabellar augmentation; and
- Temple and brow augmentation.

4.5   Injection Techniques

Dermal fillers, including HA fillers, as implied in their name, are indicated for der-mal and/or deeper plane injection. There are several different techniques of deposit-ing the filler. Serial injections of small depots of filler is probably the most com-monly used technique, especially along lin-ear regions (lip liners, nasolabial grooves). Cross-hatching or injections along 2 vec-tors at 90′ to each other works well in larger, flat areas (cheeks, tear troughs). This allows "stacking" the filler in multiple planes for a better outcome. Regardless of the tech-nique, injections are in the dermal or deeper plane with deposition of the HA

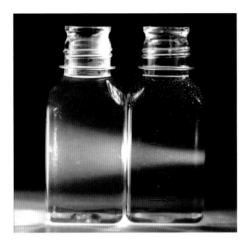

Figure 4.1 Tyndall effect; bluish hue as light is absorbed by particles.

filler in a retrograde fashion as the needle is being withdrawn. If the injection is too superficial, simply massage the filler out of the area. The phenomenon of "Tydnall effect" can occur when any particle absorbs ambient light and reflects a "bluish" color (Figure 4.1). This is applicable to an excessively superficial (epidermis) injection of HA fillers; particles of fillers will absorb light and display a blue discoloration. Patients often think this is a bruise; however, it does not resolve until the filler particles have completely dissolved. Management of the Tyndall effect will be discussed later in the chapter.

Most HA fillers have a very soft consistency and because of this, aspiration can easily be done to ensure that an intravascular injection does not occur. It is also advisable to provide local anesthesia prior to the injection for pain control (topical or intra-oral nerve blocks); this will significantly reduce patient's discomfort and can prevent inadvertent "deep" injections such as an intravascular injection due to patient's sudden movements. Some clinicians prefer to use a blunt tip cannula for injections of dermal fillers; small diameter blunt tip cannulas reduce the possibility of intravascular injections and can reduce post-operative edema. Irrespective of the injection technique or type of HA filler, placement of small increments of fillers is always advisable compared to deposition of a large amount.

4.6 Selection Process

Although most HA fillers have a gel-like consistency, there are different degrees of "viscosity" of the material. This difference is of clinical significance; for example, "softer," "less viscous" fillers may be more beneficial to use in the tear trough areas or lips where the overlying soft tissue envelope is quite thin. Conversely, for deeper planes of injection, where more volume augmentation might be necessary, more "viscous" HA fillers are indicated. Highly cross-linked HA fillers, such as *Voluma* (Allergan, Irvine, California), are indicated for cheek augmentation. Many clinicians inject in the pre-periosteal plane for these types of HA fillers. As aforementioned, all HA fillers are hydrophilic; they will induce some degree of augmentation simply due to the accumulation of water within the injection site. This phenomenon is of clinical importance as well; in areas with a thin soft tissue envelope, such as the lower lid/tear trough areas, utilization of an HA fillers with little hydrophilic properties can reduce the possibility of a "lumpy" appearance following injections. In our practice, we typically use Belotero for the tear trough region due to its paucity of hydrophilic properties.

4.7 Reversibility of HA Fillers

Perhaps one of the most important characteristics of HA fillers is the availability of an "antidote" in order to reverse unwanted side effects and complications. This is a major distinction between HA fillers and non-HA fillers; complications associated with non-HA fillers such as calcium hydroxylapatite or polymethylmethacrylate can be much more challenging to manage. Vitrase, also known as hyaluronidase (Bausch and Lomb, Rochester, New York), is an ovine-derived injectable enzyme that breaks down HA fillers in 24–48 hours. It is injected into the site of HA filler. It is imperative to remember that Vitrase will also breakdown the tissue's natural HA. This will make the surrounding skin somewhat "crapey" in appearance; this however resolves in a few days. For a novice filler clinician, having a reversal agent is a major advantage of using HA fillers over other types of fillers.

4.8 Clinical Scenarios

The following sections of this chapter will highlight specific case presentations regarding use of HA fillers for various parts of the facial region.

4.8.1 Nasolabial Grooves

Patient with moderately deep nasolabial grooves; note that cheek projection is good and filler placement along the cheeks is not necessary (Figure 4.2). In patients who have cheek deficiency, placement of fillers along this region and then augmenting the nasolabial grooves is quite beneficial. Fillers along the cheek region will elevate the soft tissue and decrease the depth of nasolabial grooves.

For this patient, 1.0 cc of Juvéderm Ultra XC was injected into bilateral nasolabial grooves after administration of intra-oral nerve block (Figures 4.2a and b). Injections were completed in a series of threading techniques along the nasolabial grooves, typically via two to three injections sites on each side.

4.8.2 Lips

Lip augmentation can be performed in two different manners. The lip proper can be augmented with HA fillers by directly injecting into the orbicularis oris muscle.

(a)
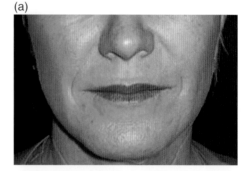
(b)
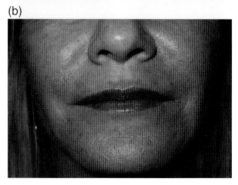

Figure 4.2 (a) Before and after (b) photos following injection of dermal fillers along nasolabial grooves.

This technique can provide large volume enhancement within the lips therefore a conservative approach is recommended. HA filler particles are placed just within the superficial aspect of the orbicularis oris muscle, just deep to the submucosal aspect of the wet part of the lips (Figure 4.3 a and b).

Other technique involves augmentation of the lip vermilion (lip liner) only without injecting directly into the lips. In this technique, the while line (vermilion) is engaged in a threading fashion. Augmentation of the lip liner area makes the lips more "pouty" without giving the appearance of unnaturally large lips (Figure 4.4 a and b).

Both augmentation cases depicted were performed using Juvéderm Ultra XC after administration of intra-oral nerve blocks.

4.8.3 Tear Troughs

Perhaps one of the most challenging regions of the face for dermal filler augmentation is the lower lid and tear trough

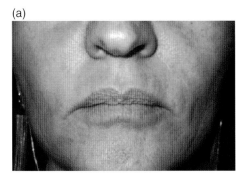

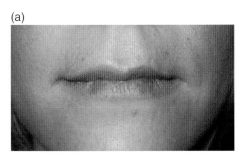

Figure 4.3 (a) Before and after (b) photos following injection of dermal fillers into the "wet" portion of the lips.

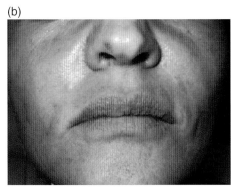

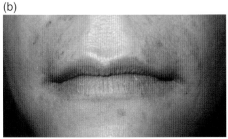

Figure 4.4 (a) Before and after (b) photos following injection of dermal fillers along the lip line (vermilion).

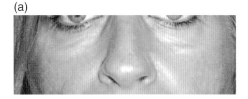

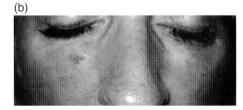

Figure 4.5 Immediate (a) before and after (b) photos following injection of dermal filler along the nasojugal areas.

areas. The lower lid is considered the thinnest skin in our body and as such, placement of HA fillers in this area must be done by an experienced practitioner. Use of HA fillers that are quite soft and do not possess strong hydrophilic activity are indicated in this area in order to avoid prolonged edema and possibility of a "lumpy" appearance. For these reason, the authors prefer to use Belotero in this region. Belotero is quite soft and does not elicit a strong hydrophilic response. Care must be taken when injecting in this region to avoid intravascular injections since vessels in this area can be quite superficial. Digital manipulation of the area right after injection of HA fillers is also recommended to blend in the results and create a smooth, homogenous result. This patient had 0.5 cc of Belotero injected in the tear trough areas in a cross-hatching technique (Figure 4.5 a and b).

4.8.4 Glabella

Certain patients will have a deep midline groove or rhytid between the right and left corrugator muscles upon contraction. This becomes especially prominent when the right and left procerus muscles have a midline separation above the nasal bridge.

(a)

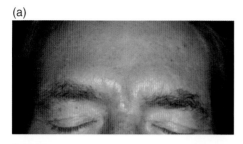

(b)

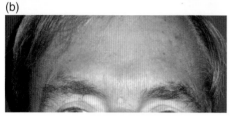

Figure 4.6 (a) Before and after (b) photos following injection of Botox and placement of dermal filler into the glabella.

These patients can benefit from augmentation of their midline groove with dermal fillers in addition to the administration of neurotoxins to relax the surrounding muscles. This patient presents with a deep midline groove/rhytid upon animation. This area was treated with 0.3 cc of Juvéderm Ultra XC in the dermal plane above the muscles and the surrounding musculature received 20 U of Botox® (Figure 4.6 a and b). It is important to place very little HA fillers in the glabella region and in the proper plane. There have been numerous reports of tissue necrosis and other periocular complications in this area due to over-injection and intravascular involvement [2–8].

4.9 Post-Injection Instructions

Patients are instructed to cleanse the injection sites with alcohol for two to three days following their appointments. Ice packs are applied immediately after the injection. No massaging is allowed for the first few days due to the soft consistency of HA fillers; excessive pressure can easily "move" the filler out of its intended place. After a week, injections sites become quite soft and supple due to "settling" of the HA fillers within the surrounding tissues. At this point, gentle massaging of any uneven area can be undertaken. Make up can certainly be applied following injection of HA fillers to camouflage any bruising. No antibiotics are indicated. If the patient has a history of perioral herpes simplex virus (HSV) infections and is undergoing perioral augmentation, anti-viral therapy such as Valtrex is initiated a day before the procedure and is continued for four to five days following. All first-time patients are asked to return to the office in two to three weeks for follow-up photographs. Patients are also instructed to call the office in case of severe discoloration (bruising vs. blanching due to vascular compromise), skin breakouts (cold sores, local tissue reaction, granulomas, etc.), and significant discomfort. These are all unusual events which deserve close attention to prevent further sequelae. In cases where a granuloma, local soft tissue reaction, or Tyndall effect does occur, application of heat and massaging are the first line of therapy. Steroid injections are helpful as well; although the threshold for injection of Vitrase in order to reverse the effects of HA fillers should be quite small (Figure 4.7).

4.10 Longevity of HA Fillers

Most HA fillers last about 9–12 months according to manufacturers' instructions. Highly cross-linked HA fillers, such as Voluma, tend to last longer (18 months), but also tend to be much more expensive compared to other types of HA fillers. In everyday clinical practice, perioral injections of HA fillers only last about five to six months due to the constant movement of the area. It is not unusual to notice HA fillers lasting longer than 9–12 months after repeated injections over time; this is probably due to

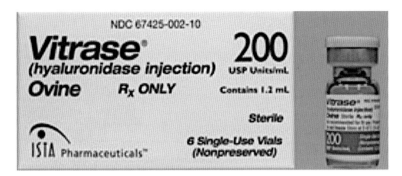

Figure 4.7 Hyaluronidase (Vitrase) used to break down HA fillers.

formation of some scar tissue at the site of injection which may act as "permanent" augmentation. Placing neurotoxins adjacent to areas that have been augmented with HA fillers can certainly prolong their longevity due to paucity of movement. All HA fillers eventually undergo a slow, dissolving process, and are eventually cleared through the liver.

4.11 Conclusion

HA dermal fillers can be a tremendously useful tool in any aesthetic practice. With proper technique and selection process, clinicians can enjoy the many benefits of these injectable fillers. HA fillers also enjoy the added benefit of having a reversal agent in cases of adverse events.

References

1 Stern, R. (2004). *Hyaluronan catabolism: a new metabolic pathway. Eur. J. Cell Biol.* 83 (7): 317–325.

2 Ferneini, E.L. and Ferneini, A.M. (2016). An overview of vascular adverse events associated with facial soft tissue fillers: recognition, prevention, and treatment. *J. Oral Maxillofac. Surg.* 74: 1630–1636.

3 Kassir, R., Kolluru, A., and Kassir, M. (2011). Extensive necrosis after injection of hyaluronic acid filler: case report and review of the literature. *J. Cosmet. Dermatol.* 10: 224.

4 Hirsch, R.J., Cohen, J.L., and Carruthers, J.D. (2007). Successful management of an unusual presentation of impending necrosis following a hyaluronic acid injection embolus and a proposed algorithm for management with hyaluronidase. *Dermatol. surg.* 33: 357.

5 Li, X., Du, L., and Lu, J.J. (2015). A novel hypothesis of visual loss secondary to cosmetic facial filler injection. *Ann. Plast. Surg.* 75: 258.

6 Beleznay, K., Carruthers, J.D., Humphrey, S. et al. (2015). Avoiding and treating blindness from fillers: a review of the world literature. *Dermatol. Surg.* 41: 1097.

7 Kim, Y.J., Kim, S.S., Song, W.K. et al. (2011). Ocular ischemia with hypotony after injection of hyaluronic acid gel. *Ophthal. Plast. Reconstr. Surg.* 27: e152.

8 Daines, S.M. and Williams, E.F. (2013). Complications associated with injectable soft tissue fillers. A 5-year retrospective review. *JAMA Facial Plast. Surg.* 15: 226.

5

Radiesse™ Calcium Hydroxylapatite Injectable Filler

Nikita Gupta[1], Onir L. Spiegel[2], and Jeffrey H. Spiegel[2,3]

[1] Department of Otolaryngology – Head and Neck Surgery, University of Kentucky Medical Center, Lexington, KY, USA
[2] The Spiegel Center, Advanced Facial Aesthetics, Newton, MA, USA
[3] Division of Facial Plastic and Reconstructive Surgery, Boston University School of Medicine, Boston, MA, USA

In December 2006 the FDA approved calcium hydroxylapatite (CaHA) as an injectable dermal filler for the correction of moderate to severe facial wrinkles and treatment for HIV lipoatrophy. Previously, it had been used safely for vocal fold augmentation, as a radiographic marker, to fill in oral/maxillofacial defects, as well as for stress urinary incontinence though in a somewhat different formulation. In 2016, it was approved for hand rejuvenation via injection into the dorsum of the hands. The material (trade name Radiesse, Merz Aesthetics) is composed of microspheres of CaHA with 25–45 μm particle sizes suspended in a carrier gel made of water, glycerin, and sodium carboxymethylcellulose.

This formulation, made of 70% carrier gel and 30% CaHA (chemical formula $Ca_{10}(PO_4)_6(OH)_2$), has an effect lasting between 10 and 14 months, with an average of 12 months [1]. Unlike the microporous formulations used as ceramics for bone reconstruction, the microsphere formulation does not support vascular ingrowth or have osteoconductive properties. The carrier gel dissipates within weeks and the microspheres remain at the site of injection until they are degraded after several months into calcium and phosphate ions excreted normally by the body. While present, they induce a fibroblastic reaction and are replaced by fibrovascular stroma [2]. The result after injection is immediate and then later sustained by neocollagen formation. As a result, Radiesse has often been considered to be a "somewhat permanent" filler, in that it induces tissue growth.

Marmur et al. initially demonstrated neocollagen formation around CaHA microspheres at six months in human skin biopsies taken after postauricular injection [3]. A canine model was used to show that CaHA injection led to endogenous collagen production with a qualitative increase in collagen formation in intradermal versus subdermal injections [4].

Berlin et al. further characterized this collagen formation with biopsies of postauricular CaHA injection in humans at six months. Hemotxylin and eosin (H&E) staining showed deposition of collagen around and infiltration into filler microspheres with a fibroblastic and a mild histiocytic tissue response. Immunohistochemical (IHC) staining confirmed Type I collagen formation and picrosirius red (PSR) staining demonstrated both Type I and Type III collagen fibers [5].

Neurotoxins and Fillers in Facial Esthetic Surgery, First Edition. Edited by Bradford M. Towne and Pushkar Mehra.
© 2019 John Wiley & Sons, Inc. Published 2019 by John Wiley & Sons, Inc.
Companion website: www.wiley.com/go/towne/neurotoxins

In a radiographic study, Carruthers et al. demonstrated that while filler material was visible on CT scans its appearance is distinct from underlying structures, it is unlikely to be confused with a pathologic finding, and it does not obscure underlying structures. The material was distinctly separate from bone and showed no osteogenesis. At the 12 month touch-up visit, preinjection CT scans showed significant decrease in the calcium deposition but a continued clinical improvement consistent with an induced neocollagen reaction in the area. This study was performed on patients obtaining injection for HIV lipoatrophy and despite the large amounts of material injected (up to 34.1 ml total), the material did not obscure underlying structures nor create new bone [6].

Multiple studies have compared the clinical results of CaHA to other dermal fillers. A pivotal trial comparing CaHA and collagen in the nasolabial folds (NLF) used a multicenter, randomized split face comparison to show superior improvement by blinded observers, similar adverse events related to injection, and decreased amount of material was needed to achieve the desired results. In the 117 patient trial, 79% of subjects had a superior result at six months (p < 0.0001) [7]. In a similar comparison between CaHA and hyaluronic acid (Restylane), CaHA was noted to be more effective at all time points up to 12 months and required 30% less material injected [8]. In a later comparison between CaHA and two hyaluronic acid products (Juvéderm Ultra and Perlane) for NLF augmentation, CaHA resulted in better patient satisfaction, longer durability, but had similar volume of material injected [9].

Adverse reactions have been described, primarily related to the injection including edema, ecchymosis, and hematoma. Of course, these particular complications are largely related to the mechanism of administration in that Radiesse must be injected. Jacovella et al. in a study for 40 patients reported a 5% adverse event rate with these reactions as well as one patient with a lip nodule that needed to be removed surgically [10]. No systemic reactions have been reported. Nodules are a particular risk of Radiesse and will be discussed further below.

5.1 Treatment in Practice

Patients who are seen for facial fillers should receive a comprehensive discussion of the relative advantages and disadvantages of each. Radiesse is often well received as a suggested filler because its primary active constituent, Calcium, is familiar to people and considered to be beneficial to overall health.

The clinician is advised to guide their patients, however, that different filler materials excel in different locations. Again, calcium is a material that patients readily associate with bone health and in our opinion Radiesse is often valuable in places where bone is being augmented, such as the malar eminences and at the superior medial aspect of the nasal labial folds near the alar groove. In both cases one can explain to the patient that we are lifting and augmenting the underlying structure with this calcium-based material. Care must be taken, however, to discuss the potential for intravascular injection with embolus and resulting ischemia.

We do not recommend this material for the tear troughs or lips as in our experience the tear troughs are too delicate an area for Radiesse, and many physicians have noted small white nodules that form in the lips after Radiesse augmentation. The hyaluronic fillers may be better used for these applications as they are softer, more readily molded, and importantly, can be reduced or eliminated fairly readily with an injection of hyaluronidase should the injection result in an undesirable appearance.

Radiesse has generally been considered to have too high a risk of visible white nodules in both of the aforementioned locations, but paradoxically it is approved for hand rejuvenation. The material can be injected deep to the skin to reduce the appearance of veins and tendons in the hands and restore the fullness of youthful hands. The injections result in moderate swelling and then benefits last typically 9–12 months.

As with all injectable fillers the injector should first conduct a thorough history specifically checking for medications such as NSAIDS, aspirin, or other blood thinners. Patients with herpes infection should be cautioned that injections can precipitate an outbreak and antiviral medications may be necessary prophylactically in advance of and following the injection.

Bruising is a potential side effect of any injection and Radiesse treatments are no exception. Blunt tip micro cannulas may reduce the incidence of bruising and can reduce another potential dangerous side effect of injectables, the inadvertent injection of the material into an intravascular space. Radiesse, as a particulate injectable, has a risk of embolization if inadvertently injected in this fashion and complications such as vision loss or even blindness could occur in certain locations.

Radiesse comes in two formulations including the standard preparation and a "+" formation that includes lidocaine. Prior to the introduction of this version physicians would commonly mix the 1.5 cc size Radiesse with 0.3 cc of 1% lidocaine with epinephrine and the 0.8 cc size with 0.15 cc of this same anesthetic preparation. Mixing was done with a standard two syringe mixing valve being certain to prevent air from being introduced into the mixture.

Radiesse+™ or the original formulation mixed with lidocaine are relatively comfortable for injection through a 27 gauge needle. Injection should be done deep to the dermis to prevent visible white lines or nodules. The material can be placed into the subcutaneous fat or directly on or near the periosteum without stimulating bony growth. In the senior author's experience

injections are well tolerated and regional or local nerve blocks are not necessary. Injection can be done essentially to complete correction to prevent a period of time with excess filling, however the carrier carboxymethylcellulose is cleared by the body relatively quickly and patient's should expect a correction that is less than what they see in the initial post-injection period.

Different locations should be treated with specific injection techniques. The senior author prefers a bolus technique at the superior medial aspect of the nasolabial fold in order to elevate the skin at this area and correct the volume loss associated with aging in this area. A similar technique is done for the malar eminence with the anterior flattening being the key focus of the correction.

Tear troughs are not recommended for treatment in general, though if they were to be addressed only a small amount of filler would be used deep along the periosteum.

Lip injections are not recommended as many authors have noted that the injection, even if smoothly administered, can clump into small white visible nodules that may need to be removed. The sharp edge of a 19 gauge needle can be used to scoop these nodules out of the lip with minimal disruption of the surrounding tissues in many cases.

Marionette lines can be injected best by a transverse incision perpendicular to the vector of the fold along its superior aspect. This injection forms something of a "bar" that supports the fold and provides good resolution. Direct bolus injection in this area can otherwise result in a ball of filler that distends the mucosa of the mouth and creates a palpable mass that patients find disconcerting.

Radiesse is also useful for what is commonly called nonsurgical rhinoplasty. Nasal irregularities and twists can occasionally be corrected by filling in the concave area with Radiesse deep along the nasal bones or cartilages.

This can create the illusion of a straight nose by making the external skin more symmetrically draped. Similarly nasal irregularities such as a deep radix can be improved with Radiesse though great caution must be taken to prevent intravascular injection of the material with the aforementioned risks of embolization and complications.

The risk of intravascular injection should be stressed for this particulate injectable material. Ischemia can form also from compression of a blood vessel such as the angular artery. Treatment can be difficult as the material cannot be readily dissolved in the way that hyaluronic filers can be rapidly eliminated. Nitro paste, steroids, and other treatments may be required to address such a complication.

In summary, Radiesse is a reliable filler that patients are comfortable with and consider to be a natural volumizing option that is consistent with prevailing attitudes regarding calcium as a healthy mineral. Micro cannula injection may reduce the risk of complications and the material is approved for use in the hands, though it should be avoided in the lips.

References

1 Graivier, M.H., Bass, L.S., Busso, M. et al. (2007 Nov). Calcium hydroxylapatite (Radiesse) for correction of the mid- and lower face: consensus recommendations. *Plast. Reconstr. Surg.* 120 (6 Suppl): 55S–66S.

2 Berlin, A.L., Hussain, M., and Goldberg, D.J. (2008 Jun). Calcium hydroxylapatite filler for facial rejuvenation: a histologic and immunohistochemical analysis. *Dermatol. Surg.* 34 (Suppl 1): S64–S567.

3 Marmur, E.S., Phelps, R., and Goldberg, D.J. (2004 Dec). Clinical, histologic and electron microscopic findings after injection of a calcium hydroxylapatite filler. *J. Cosmet. Laser Ther.* 6 (4): 223–226.

4 Coleman, K.M., Voigts, R., DeVore, D.P. et al. (2008 Jun). Neocollagenesis after injection of calcium hydroxylapatite composition in a canine model. *Dermatol. Surg.* 34 (Suppl 1): S53–S55.

5 Berlin, A.L., Hussain, M., and Goldberg, D.J. (2008 Jun). Calcium hydroxylapatite filler for facial rejuvenation: a histologic and immunohistochemical analysis. *Dermatol. Surg.* 34 (Suppl 1): S64–S567.

6 Carruthers, A., Liebeskind, M., Carruthers, J. et al. (2008 Jun). Radiographic and computed tomographic studies of calcium hydroxylapatite for treatment of HIV-associated facial lipoatrophy and correction of nasolabial folds. *Dermatol. Surg.* 34 (Suppl 1): S78–S84.

7 Smith, S., Busso, M., McClaren, M. et al. (2007 Dec). A randomized, bilateral, prospective comparison of calcium hydroxylapatite microspheres versus human-based collagen for the correction of nasolabial folds. *Dermatol. Surg.* 33 (Suppl 2): S112–S121; discussion S121.

8 Moers-Carpi, M.M. and Tufet, J.O. (2008 Feb). Calcium hydroxylapatite versus nonanimal stabilized hyaluronic acid for the correction of nasolabial folds: a 12-month, multicenter, prospective, randomized, controlled, split-face trial. *Dermatol. Surg.* 34 (2): 210–215.

9 Moers-Carpi, M., Vogt, S., Santos, B.M. et al. (2007 Dec). A multicenter, randomized trial comparing calcium hydroxylapatite to two hyaluronic acids for treatment of nasolabial folds. *Dermatol. Surg.* 33 (Suppl 2): S144–S151.

10 Jacovella, P.F., Peiretti, C.B., Cunille, D. et al. (2006 Sep). Long-lasting results with hydroxylapatite (Radiesse) facial filler. *Plast. Reconstr. Surg.* 118 (3 Suppl): 15S–21S.

6

Pearls and Pitfalls of Neurotoxins and Facial Fillers

Raffi Der Sarkissian

Boston Facial Plastic Surgery, Boston, MA, USA
Division of Facial Plastic Surgery, Boston University School of Medicine, Boston, MA, USA
Division of Facial Plastic Surgery, Massachusetts Eye and Ear Infirmary, Boston, MA, USA

6.1 Pearls and Pitfalls in Neurotoxin Use

Success in the use of neurotoxins and fillers in the face relies on accurate analysis of the area(s) to be treated and correct application of the appropriate techniques for correction of each proposed area. It is imperative to determine if aging changes are related to textural changes in the skin itself, lines and furrows created by repetitive muscle movement, loss of elasticity with resultant skin and soft tissue ptosis, facial volume loss or redistribution or a combination of these elements. If upon analysis, it is felt that the lines and wrinkles are a result of over activity of certain facial muscles, the benefits of neurotoxins have been well documented [1]. Following certain technical "pearls of wisdom" can mean the difference between a good and an excellent result and can minimize the possibility of an adverse result.

6.2 Neurotoxin Preparation and Storage

Commercially available neurotoxins (Onabotulinum toxin A, Abobotulinum toxin A and Incobotulinum toxin A) are provided in a vacuum dried or lyophilized state. Each requires reconstitution with injectable saline (0.9% sodium chloride). The type of diluent used has been debated with most companies recommending the use of preservative-free saline while some practitioners preferring preserved saline. As alcohol is used as a preservative in saline, dilution with preserved saline may create more burning on injection. Some practitioners propose the opposite to be true and feel the alcohol acts as an anesthetic resulting in less pain. Preservative-free saline is this author's preference for dilution.

While diluting the product, it is imperative to know the concentration of the neurotoxin and attempt to reliably duplicate the required dilution for each vial. The volume used for dilution is not as critical as knowledge of the number of units per unit volume of diluted product (1–5 ml dilutions have been described). The benefit of lower-volume dilution with higher concentration of toxin is the ability to use smaller volumes of injectate per site with theoretically less pain on injection and a more focused effect. Conversely, a higher volume dilution will allow the practitioner a more widespread distribution of an equivalent number of units of toxin. I have found a 3 ml dilution to be ideal, yielding a concentration of 3.3 Onabotulinum toxin units per 0.1 ml aliquot. Equally important is knowledge of the relative strengths of the commercially available products. As most initial studies of the efficacy of neurotoxins were conducted with Onabotulinum toxin (Botox), this is generally considered as the "standard" strength of toxin.

Conversion ratios have been developed for Abobotulinum toxin A (Dysport) and Incobotulinum A (Xeomin) as follows:

1 Onabotulinum toxin unit = 2.5–3.0 Abobotulinum toxin units
1 Onabotulinum toxin unit = 1.0–1.5 Incobotulinum toxin units

6.3 Choice of Syringes and Needles

There are a number of personal preferences in syringe and needle types for injection of neurotoxins. Most authors agree a small volume syringe 0.3–1.0 ml is ideal. Fixed needle syringes have the advantage of ease of use, however, in drawing up toxin the needles tend to dull easily (Figure 6.1).

Syringes with detachable needles allow changing of needles to fit the practitioners' preference. Syringes that have a plunger that extends into the hub have the advantage of not wasting any product (Figure 6.2).

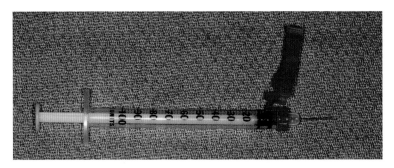

Figure 6.1 Fixed needle syringes offer the convenience of not needing to change needles. However, if the needle dulls during injection it cannot be changed, thus requiring transfer of toxin to another syringe, which causes associated toxin waste.

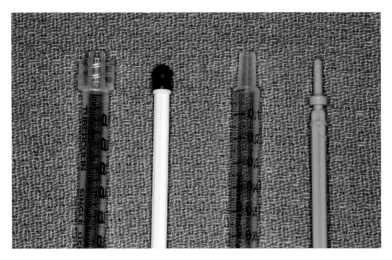

Figure 6.2 The plunger of the syringe on the right extends into the hub of the syringe assuring only a very small volume of toxin is wasted.

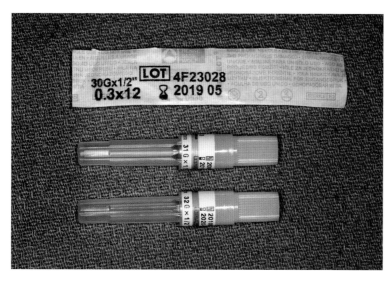

Figure 6.3 Very fine gauge needles can help minimize pain associated with toxin injections.

Drawing up toxin can be performed with a larger gauge needle (25–20 gauge) and injection can be performed with a finer gauge needle (33–30 gauge). Be aware that these finer needles are generally less traumatic, however, they do dull easily and if a number of injections will be performed, changing the needle is recommended. (Figure 6.3)

6.4 Basic Injection Principles

Placing needles in a patient's forehead, around their eyes and in other anatomic sites around the face can induce fear, anxiety, and pain. Patients will often comment on injections being "painful," "rushed," "unpleasant" or causing significant post-injection discomfort and/or bruising. Although bruising is possible even in the hands of the most skilled clinicians, the following techniques can minimize some negative effects and offer patients a more comfortable experience.

1) Verbalize what to expect and where to expect the pain. "You will feel a pinch between the brows followed by a little burning."

2) Counting before injection helps patients anticipate the pain and not move reflexively during the injection.

3) Use the smallest gauge needle and replace the needle as needed when dull.

4) Consider using a topical anesthetic or pretreating with ice in extremely sensitive patients.

5) Use digital pressure prior to injection to alleviate the discomfort in sensitive patients.

6) Stretching the skin between the fingers allows the needle to penetrate more easily. Think of trying to sew fabric that is loose versus fabric that is stretched taught.

7) Enter the skin tangentially. This helps to avoid contacting the underlying bone, particularly in areas of thin skin. Additionally, when the needle is placed sub-dermally at an angle, it becomes easier to enter the subcutaneous muscle and deliver a bolus of toxin rather than entering vertically into relatively thin muscles with less chance of accuracy in toxin delivery. Think of laminated sheets of paper and the middle sheets of paper need to be saturated

with liquid. Entering at an angle makes this exercise easier.

8) Always look for obvious surface vasculature and attempt to avoid penetrating a vessel. Entering the skin tangentially can help here as well as the needle can be oriented away from any visible vessel.

9) Treat muscles diffusely with small aliquots of toxin in multiple locations rather than larger boluses with the "expectation" that the toxin will diffuse into the target muscle. This leads to more accurate patterns of chemodenervation, minimizes risk of untoward results from diffusion of product away from the target muscle and minimizes the risk of incomplete treatment of a muscle group and its related pattern of rhytids.

10) Always treat one entire muscle group at a time, starting on one side and treating the contralateral side with the same pattern of injection and the same dose of toxin. For example, treat the procerus in the midline of the glabella followed by the right medial corrugator, the left medial corrugator, the right mid corrugator, left mid corrugator, right distal (lateral) corrugator, and left distal (lateral) corrugator. In so doing, each side of the muscle will have the same injection sites along the muscle and the same dose and treatments with a higher chance of yielding symmetric results.

11) After injection, apply digital pressure to the injection site in the direction you would like the toxin to diffuse and away from structure you are trying to avoid. This not only helps diffuse the toxin into the muscle more quickly but limits any potential bruising that might occur.

12) Studies have shown reconstituted neurotoxins to maintain activity up to two weeks after reconstitution. It is recommended, however, to use toxins soon after reconstitution, ideally within the same calendar day.

13) If storing reconstituted neurotoxin, do not freeze the product as this has been noted to decrease activity, possibly by damaging the carrier protein.

14) Store the lyophilized product between 2 and 8 °C (36–46 °F)

6.5 Specific Injection Pearls Based on Injection Site

6.5.1 Glabellar Techniques

Obliquely oriented "inverted V shaped" lines are a result of contraction of the paired corrugator supercilii muscles. Horizontally oriented lines across the glabella are a result of contraction of the midline procerus muscle.

The procerus muscle originates on the nasal bone and attaches to the skin of the glabella or low midline forehead [2]. Having patients animate by asking them to "lower their brow" or create an "angry look" will help assess the vertical height of the muscle and help guide the number of injections required. Generally two injections will suffice in this area. The more inferior injection is placed somewhat more deeply and the superior injection more superficially to target the muscle depth more accurately. Small doses in the range of 3–10 Onabotulinum toxin units are usually enough to control the horizontal rhytids.

The corrugator supercilii muscles originate on the supraorbital ridge of the frontal bone and insert onto the skin above the brow generally anywhere between the root of the brow and the midbrow [3]. In treating this area, it is imperative to have the patient create an "angry look" and assess the length of the corrugator. Assessment of the length and bulk of the muscle will help with decisions about dose required and how many injections will be required to adequately decrease

Figure 6.4 (a) Horizontally oriented corrugator supercilii muscle. Injections 1–4 are placed deeper. Sites 7 and 8 are optional only if muscle length extends laterally. The more medial injections are placed deeply, the more lateral superficially. (b) Vertically/obliquely oriented corrugator supercilii muscle. Injections 1–4 are placed deeply, 5 and 6 more superficially.

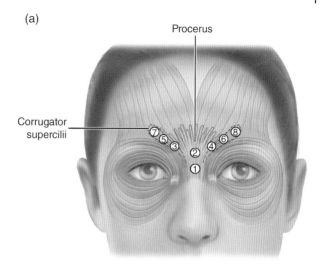

(a)

Procerus

Corrugator supercilii

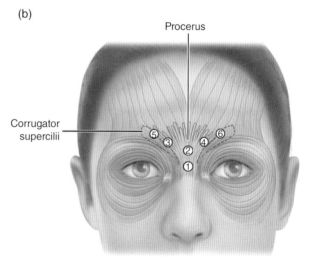

(b)

Procerus

Corrugator supercilii

movement in the area and improve the appearance of the oblique furrows. At least two points of injection are required on each side. A muscle treated at only a single point can still contract medially or laterally to the point of injection resulting in post injection lines proximal or distal to the pre-treatment furrows.

Generally three to four points of injection are recommended on each side based on the length of the muscle. The medial injections should be slightly deeper as the muscle originates on the bone and moving laterally, the injections should be more superficial targeting the muscle attachments to the skin (Figures 6.4a and 6.4b).

Injections in the suprabrow region should always be placed at least 1 cm above the supraorbital rim. Placement of the injector's thumb on the rim helps to respect this anatomic requirement and also increases the resistance to flow of injectate to prevent diffusion to the levator palpebrae muscle minimizing the risk of upper eyelid ptosis.

On an average, approximately 15–30 Onabotulinum toxin A units are generally required to adequately treat the corrugator supercilii muscles and minimize glabellar oblique furrows.

Both the midline procerus and paired corrugators are depressors of the medial brow and medially constrict the brows. As such, successful treatment of this area should yield a "relaxation" of the space between the brows and relative elevation of the root of the brow.

As the muscles in this area are associated with expressions of anger, they are, from an evolutionary standpoint, required for "survival" and hence can be quite strong. Under correction, even with adequate doses of toxin are not uncommon. It is important to remind first-time-treatment patients that it may require retreating the area at four month intervals for two or three additional sessions to achieve more significant relaxation of the rhytids. In difficult-to-treat glabellar muscles, or in patients with grooves deeply "etched" into the skin, small volumes of low density fillers can help soften the appearance of horizontal or oblique grooves or furrows.

6.5.2 Forehead Techniques

Horizontal lines in the forehead are a result of contraction of the paired frontalis muscles. The frontalis originates from the galea aponeurotica at the level of the frontal hairline. Distally, the muscle attaches to the skin of the brows [2]. Evaluation of the cause of the horizontal furrows is important in treating the forehead region. Some patients have lines simply as a result of frontalis hyperactivity and excess facial animation. More commonly, horizontal lines are a result of chronic elevation of an anatomically low brow or pseudo ptosis or true ptosis of the upper eyelids. As the frontalis is the only true elevator of the brow, proper evaluation of the upper third of the face in repose and in animation is an absolute requirement before treating with neurotoxins. Failure to identify ptosis of the brow or upper eyelids can result in inability to raise the brows and yield an undesirable result.

The female brow should lie above the superior bony orbital rim, the male brow should be at or above the rim. The female brow should have a peak somewhere between the lateral limbus of the iris and the lateral canthus. The male brow tends to remain more horizontal along its length. Ideally the tail of the brow should sit above the position of the root of the brow. When treating the forehead, it is important to treat the entire frontalis muscle. Inadequate treatment of the lateral frontalis can lead to unopposed action of the lateral part of the muscle yielding an abnormally peaked lateral brow.

Although anatomically, there is frequently a gap in the midline between the left and right sided frontalis, treatment should include injections at or near the midline of the forehead to avoid a residual rhytid centrally in an otherwise smooth forehead If the frontalis is noted to extend up to the level of the hairline, it is important to have the injections extend superiorly to the uppermost extent of the muscle. Failure to do so may result in a deep furrow at or just below the hairline which is clearly visible particularly when the remaining forehead is rendered smooth with neurotoxin.

As with glabellar injections, one should not inject within 1 cm of the supraorbital rim [4]. Along the lateral brow, staying above this 1 cm margin can occasionally result in a residual crescent shaped furrow just above the brow that may be bothersome to some patients. Extreme caution should be exercised in further treatment to this area and the risk of lateral brow ptosis as compared with the benefit of further reduction in this furrow should be discussed with each individual patient. Generally, a small remaining

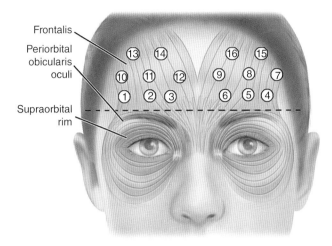

Figure 6.5 In order to avoid brow ptosis, injections are started 2–3 cm above the orbital rim. Treatment of the lateral frontalis 1,4,7,10 will decrease the chance of excessively elevated lateral brow. Eliminating injections 1 and 4 will create a lift of the lateral brow in patients who desire a temporal brow elevation. Injections 3, 6, 9, and 12 at or near the midline will reduce the chance of leaving a solitary midline rhytid. Injections 13–16 are optional but should be considered in patients who have rhytids at or near the hairline on animation.

lateral brow rhytid is desirable as compared with lateral brow ptosis and lateral canthal hooding.

In patients desiring elevation of the lateral brow, a central "V" shaped pattern of injection can be considered to maintain the position of the central and medial brow while allowing the lateral frontalis to elevate the lateral brow. This pattern of injection may take some trial and error in achieving the ideal amount of lateral lift [5]. Precise documentation of the locations injected and the doses used is imperative.

Although some patients may have a very dominant deep mid forehead furrow and would benefit from a single "row" of injections directly above or below the deep line, most patients have better results with at least two parallel rows of injection with more diffuse denervation of the muscle (Figure 6.5).

As the frontalis is a very superficial muscle, small boluses of toxin should be injected subcutaneously. Here the tangential orientation of the needle is preferred to a more vertical injection technique.

In general, 15–30 units of Onabotulinum toxin A are adequate for treatment of the forehead. Overtreatment or treatment too close to the brow complex may lead to brow ptosis and eyelid pseudo ptosis. The "heaviness" associated with overtreatment starts to improve three to four weeks after treatment as some frontalis muscle fibers begin to work. It is always best to "ease" into treatment when chemodenervating the frontalis, keeping in mind one can always add a few more units or treat another site for under correction but overcorrection cannot be improved until the toxin effect reverses.

6.5.3 Periorbital Techniques

Radial periorbital lines are a result of contracture of the orbital portion of the orbicularis oculi muscle. These should not be confused with more inferior periorbital rhytids associated with contraction of the deeper zygomaticus major muscle. The former can be effectively treated with chemodenervation; the latter cannot and attempts to do so may yield decreased

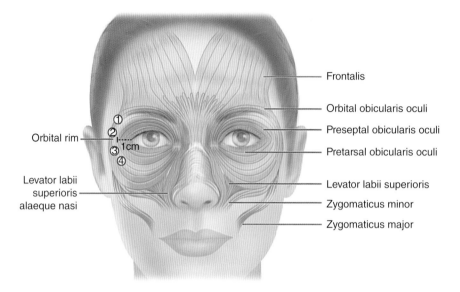

Figure 6.6 Injections should be superficial and at least 1 cm lateral to the lateral orbital rim. Injection 4 is optional. Note the proximity of this injection to the head of the zygomaticus major muscle which lies deep to the orbicularis.

lateral commissure elevation and potential distortion of the smile.

A clinical method of differentiating between lines resulting from orbicularis oculi contracture and zygomaticus contracture is to have the patient close the eyes tightly, to illustrate lines caused by the orbicularis, and to smile to show lines caused by zygomaticus contracture. It is helpful to have patients close one eye while looking in a mirror to show the periorbital lines that are effectively treated with neurotoxin. Having them smile will illustrate lines not amenable to treatment.

Injections should be very superficial as the orbicularis lies directly under the thin periorbital skin and superficial to the proximal zygomaticus major muscle. Too deep of an injection can impair zygomatic muscle function. Injections should be 1 cm lateral to the bony rim to avoid diffusion to the levator palpebrae superioris. The periorbital area is highly vascular. Oftentimes, with proper illumination, the superficial vessels are visible and care must be taken to avoid injury. Patients are always warned about the possibility of bruising which is slightly higher in this area than other sites on the face.

Two to four injection are placed starting at about the level of the lateral brow and ending along a vertical line drawn approximately 1 cm below the lateral canthus. Occasionally, an additional injection can be placed slightly medial to this plumb line with caution given to staying superficial and monitoring for any lid retrusion resulting from the medial placement of toxin (Figure 6.6).

Generally speaking, 6–20 units of Onabotulinum toxin A total are injected. As the orbital orbicularis is a lateral depressor of the brow, treatment of this muscle results in a slight elevation of the lateral brow. In patients desiring lateral brow elevation, this technique, combined with not treating the lateral frontalis, is quite effective. Combining this technique with treating the corrugator supercilii and procerus (depressors of the medial brow) can effectively result in an overall brow position elevation.

6.5.4 Treatment of Bunny Lines

Bunny lines are created across the nasal sidewall and dorsum as a function of contraction of the nasalis muscle and the procerus. The area is not commonly treated unless patients are bothered by the appearance or if the force of the contraction significantly depresses the medial brow. As with other anatomic injections of neurotoxins, the muscle should be localized by having the patient "sniff" or be asked to wrinkle their nose "like a rabbit." The muscle is superficial just beneath the relatively thin nasal sidewall/dorsal skin. Generally, one to three injections of one to three units each are adequate to suppress excess nasalis activity (Figure 6.7).

Care must be taken to not inject the more laterally based levator labii superioris alaeque nasi muscles which are lip elevators. Diffusion into or direct injection into the levator labii may result in lip ptosis or asymmetric elevation of the lip on smiling.

6.5.5 Depressor Anguli Oris Techniques

The depressor anguli oris (DAO) is responsible for pulling down the lateral commissure of the lip. Treatment of the DAO with neurotoxin will serve to weaken this function and allow for relatively unopposed zygomaticus major muscle contraction resulting in elevation of the corners of the mouth.

Care must be taken not to inject the more medial depressor labii or mentalis muscles [2]. Doing so can create a distorted smile or asymmetry during speech. The patient is asked to frown or "show their lower teeth." If the belly of the muscle is visible or palpable, a single injection of two to five units is made into the muscle. If the muscle is not apparent on animation, the injection can be made approximately 1 cm superior to the mandibular border just lateral to the point of attachment of the mandibular ligament. If any jowling is present, this point is usually just at the anterior border of the jowl. Anatomically, to avoid treatment of the more medial muscles, injections should be placed at least 1 cm lateral and 1 cm inferior to the oral commissure (Figure 6.8).

6.5.6 Perioral Techniques

Radial wrinkles around the mouth related to puckering, drinking through a

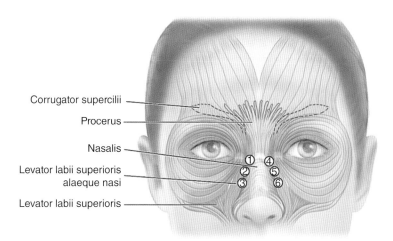

Corrugator supercilii
Procerus
Nasalis
Levator labii superioris alaeque nasi
Levator labii superioris

Figure 6.7 Injection for "bunny line" contraction of transverse portion of the nasalis muscle, Injections 1, 2, 4, and 5 are generally adequate for correction. Injections 3 and 6 are optional and only used when the furrows are very deep. Treatment should include the inferior procerus.

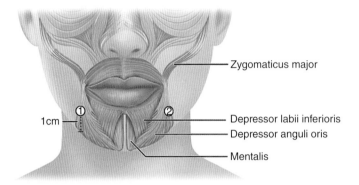

Figure 6.8 Preferred injection site for the DAO muscle. 1 cm above the mandibular border, just lateral to a vertical line dropped from the lateral commissure.

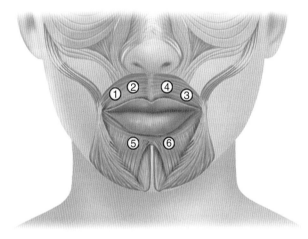

Figure 6.9 Injection for radial lines around the lips. Lines are generally more apparent on the upper lip. Injections 5 and 6 are beneficial in patients with prominent lower lip lines as well.

straw and, most commonly, smoking are amenable to treatment with very small doses of neurotoxin. Sphincteric contraction of the orbicularis oris muscle is responsible for the perioral lines. Injection of small aliquots of neurotoxin (one to two units per injection) in two to four positions along the upper and lower lip can be effective in "softening" the lines (Figure 6.9). Patients are always warned that even with these small doses, there may be some changes in articulation, the "posture" of the upper or lower lip and that drinking through a straw may be affected. Larger doses can result in

significant smile asymmetry and upper or lower lip ptosis. Rather than risking asymmetry or issues with puckering during pursing the lips or drinking, a combination of very low dose neurotoxin treatment in combination with low density fillers or fillers alone may be safer alternatives.

6.5.7 Levator Labii Superioris alaeque Nasi

Over activity of the levator labii superioris alaeque nasi can result in excess elevation of the upper lip resulting in a "gummy smile." The muscle originates on the

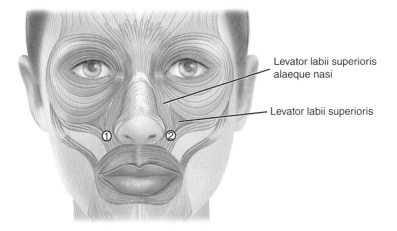

Levator labii superioris alaeque nasi

Levator labii superioris

Figure 6.10 Single injection of the inferior aspect of the levator labii superioris alaeque nasi will decrease lip elevation with smiling.

anterior surface of the maxilla and attaches to the skin above the vermilion in line with the alar base. Single, small dose injections (one to two units) at the inferior border of the muscle above the orbicularis oris help decrease contraction of the muscle and may reduce the gummy smile appearance (Figure 6.10).

Care should be taken not to overcorrect to avoid lip ptosis and to not inject into the orbicularis oris muscle itself which may distort the smile.

6.5.8 Techniques for Chin Dimpling

"Peu d'orange" or dimpling of the skin of the chin can be seen in patients with hyperactive mentalis muscles. The mentalis is a central depressor of the lower lip which attaches to the skin of the lower lip and creates the labiomental groove. Neurotoxin injected into the mentalis can help relax the muscle and soften the dimpled appearance of the chin. Each muscle is injected with four to eight units along two to four vertically oriented injection sites. Injections are kept low, close to the mental border to avoid inadvertent treatment of the orbicularis oris muscle, which can result in lower lip ptosis (Figure 6.11).

6.5.9 Treatment of Platysmal Bands

The platysma is a flat muscle that inserts onto the clavicle and acromion inferiorly and onto the anterior inferior aspect of the mentum and posteriorly over the mandible. Below the hyoid, the muscles exist as two separate paired muscles while superiorly, the muscle tends to decussate before insertion of the mandible [2]. In youth, the paired muscle bands tend to be more closely aligned in the midline. As a function of age, the muscle bands lateralize and the anterior edge of the muscles can create "banding." In simple ptosis of the muscle, surgical correction is the most effective way to eliminate the bands [6].

In some patients, banding can occur because of hyperactivity of the platysma muscle. This is generally more common in thinner patients and in patients who have had submental liposuction or lipectomy exposing the hyperfunctional bands. In these patients, treatment with neurotoxin can be effective in flattening the bands.

Asking the patient to grimace or "show their lower teeth" will accentuate the muscle bands. Grasping the anterior edge of the muscle will allow better localization of the muscle for injection. Beginning at least 2 cm below the border of the

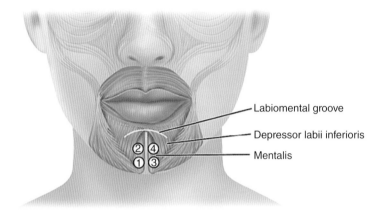

Figure 6.11 1–4 injections are performed deeply into the body of the mentalis muscle. Avoid injecting laterally into the depressor labii muscle. Avoid injecting above the labiomental groove.

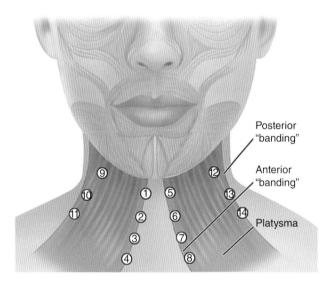

Figure 6.12 Injections 1–3 and 5–7 are most important in addressing the anterior bands. Injections 4 and 8 may be required if the banding extends low in the neck. Injections 9–14 are only necessary if there are prominent posterior bands.

mandible, two to four units are injected in three or four positions along the entire length of the muscle (Figure 6.12).

Posterior/lateral bands, if present, can be treated in a similar fashion. Extreme caution should be exercised in not injecting deep to the platysma to avoid weakening deeper cervical muscles. Over injection of this area has been associated with dysphagia, voice change and aspiration.

6.5.10 Treatment for Masseter Hypertrophy

The masseter muscle originates along the zygomatic arch and onto the body and ramus of the mandibular angle. Overactivity of the masseter muscle as seen in habitual clenching or bruxism can lead to hypertrophy of the muscle. Certain individuals may have hypertrophic muscle even in the absence of overactivity. In either

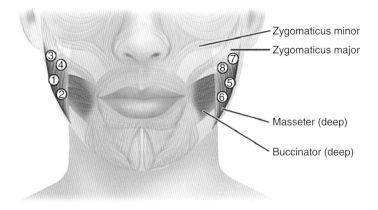

Zygomaticus minor
Zygomaticus major

Masseter (deep)

Buccinator (deep)

Figure 6.13 Injection of the masseter is preferred deep into the muscle bulk at 2–4 points on each side. Smaller doses and fewer injection points doses are required in mild hypertrophy while higher doses in a more diffuse distribution pattern may be required for more significant muscle enlargement. Results may take four to six weeks and generally a series of 2–3 injections may be required.

case, although excess bigonial width may be attractive with certain facial shapes, ethnic groups, or male gender patients, the presence of an enlarged masseter may impart an overly square look to the face. Neurotoxins are effective in temporarily decreasing the bulk and action of the muscle [7].

With one finger placed anterior to the muscle and a second at the angle of the mandible, the patient is asked to clench down to contract the masseter. With the patient continuing to clench down, injections of three to five units are made in two to four different positions along the muscle. Generally, 10–20 units are used depending on the bulk of the muscle. As the muscle attaches to bone and is relatively thick, the injections should be placed deeply and ideally into the middle of the muscle belly. The injections should remain inferior and posterior into the muscle to avoid diffusion superiorly or anteriorly into the muscles of facial expression (Figure 6.13).

6.6 Neurotoxin Complications

Fortunately, the cosmetic use of neurotoxins is relatively safe and no reports of permanent adverse reactions directly related to the toxin have, to our knowledge, been documented [8]. The most common complications are related to local diffusion to adjacent muscles or improper injection of the toxin. Careful injection with an understanding that the injectate can diffuse 1–3 cm is imperative. Bruising, swelling, pain, and erythema are common general side effects of neurotoxin injection. Careful injection techniques using small gauge needles, small aliquots of injectate and local pressure can significantly reduce the bruising and swelling. Application of ice prior to injection mitigates the pain of injection and can help vasoconstrict vessels to decrease bruising.

Patients on anticoagulants should be advised they may have more significant bruising on injection. For anticoagulated patients who are not willing to accept this possibility, injections should be avoided. Reactions such as headache, nausea, flu-like symptoms, rash, pruritis, and respiratory tract infections have been reported. However, in controlled studies, the incidence of these has not been statistically significant versus placebo controls [9]. Ptosis of the brow is the most significant complication of treating the forehead. As the frontalis is the sole elevator of the brows, overtreatment of the brow, particularly in the distal 2–4 cm near the brow can result in brow ptosis. Patients with anatomically low riding brows should not be treated along the forehead or, should only be treated along the proximal, superior-most portion of the frontalis muscle.

Inadequate injection of the lateral aspect of the frontalis muscle can lead to unopposed action of the lateral frontalis and an abnormally elevated lateral brow imparting an angry look to the face sometimes referred to as the "Jack Nicholson" or "Dr. Spock" look. Small doses of toxin delivered to the lateral frontalis can correct this abnormal elevation. Diffusion of neurotoxin to the levator palpebrae superioris, from glabellar or forehead injections, can result in ptosis of the eyelid. Should this occur, alpha adrenergic ophthalmic drops (e.g. neosynephrine hydrochloride 2.5% or Iopidine) can be used to stimulate Muller's muscle and can raise a ptotic eyelid up to 2 mm. Generally, correction of the ptosis to a level adequate enough to minimize the asymmetry occurs within two to four weeks.

In treating the periorbital area, bruising is the most common complication. Based on the vascularity of the skin around the eye, this can be quite significant. Avoidance by careful examination for obvious surface vessels is imperative. Diffusion into the preseptal or pretarsal component of the orbicularis oculi muscle can lead to reduction in blinking and poor eye closure. Lubrication of the eye during the day with drops, and use of ophthalmic ointment with or without taping the eye shut at night may be required. Diffusion of toxin or direct injection into the lower lid pretarsal or preseptal orbicularis to increase the palpebral fissure width can lead to ectropion and keratoconjunctivitis sicca. The risk of ectropion is higher in patients with poor lower lid tone or those who have had previous eyelid surgery.

Diffusion into the superior zygomaticus major muscle while trying to reduce the appearance of crow's feet can result in an asymmetric smile [10]. Anatomically, the orbicularis oculi is located subcutaneously while the zygomaticus is deeper, attaching to the lateral orbital rim. Distortion of the smile can persist for four to six weeks post injection. Perioral injections and their complications have been discussed, most commonly involving distortion of the smile, difficulty with whistling or drinking through a straw and potential oral incompetence. Careful knowledge of the target muscle anatomy can help avoid these unwanted sequelae.

With diffusion into the more laterally based levator labii superioris alaeque nasi distortion of the lip contour, smile, or functional deficits around the lips and mouth can occur with treatment of bunny lines.

Injection of the neck with diffusion into the deeper cervical muscles can lead to dysphagia, voice change, or aspiration. The dysphagia and voice change may persist for two to four weeks. Any patient with known or suspected aspiration, should be referred for a swallowing evaluation and advised on techniques of preventing aspiration until the muscle blockade reverses.

6.7 Cosmetic Facial Fillers: Pearls and Pitfalls

Definitions of various aging-related changes of the face are quite variable and inconsistent. Practitioners often use terms such as folds, furrows, and grooves interchangeably and incorrectly. Generally, in describing a "line" in the face, the terminology should reflect the anatomic location and whether the line is a "deficit" between anatomic subunits (a groove) or a fullness above or below the "deficit" (a fold).

It is also imperative to determine if the lines or grooves are within the substance of the skin (textural), due to overall loss of elasticity of the skin creating folds and grooves related to skin redundancy, or due to a "deflation" phenomenon resulting from loss of facial fat and soft tissue support.

Textural changes might be best treated with resurfacing techniques with or without the addition of fine line facial fillers. Redundant skin and soft tissue ptosis might be most amenable to treatment with surgical "resuspension" with post-operative use of fillers as needed. Significant volume loss in the face may be treated with replacement of facial volume or may benefit from combined treatments [11].

This analysis will allow the practitioner to use the most effective treatment available to improve the aesthetic deficit. If facial fillers will be considered, deciding which product is best suited for correction and the appropriate anatomic location for injection are the essential determinants of success [12].

As such, fillers can be generally classified as follows:

Hyaluronic acid fillers

Thin, low viscosity, lower G-prime value
    Restylane Silk
    Restylane Refyne
    Juvederm Volbella
    Juvederm Ultra
    Belotero

Medium thickness, intermediate viscosity and G-prime
    Restylane
    Restylane Defyne
    Juvederm Ultra Plus
    Juvederm Vollure

Thick, denser viscosity, higher G-prime
    Restylane Lyft
    Juvederm Voluma

Filler/Collagen inducer
    Calcium hydroxylapatite (Radiesse)

Collegen inducers
    Poly-L-lactic acid (Sculptra)

Permanent Fillers
    Polymethylmethacrylate (Artefill)*
    Injectable Silicone*
    Polyacrylamide Gel*

Knowledge of the nuances of each filler comes with studying the science behind

---

* Author has no experience with injectable polymethylmethacrylate, silicone or polyacrylamide gel, with the exception of surgical removal of these products injected elsewhere.

each of the products, reviewing the experience of other practitioners and most importantly, personal experience. For example, various hyaluronic acid (HA) products have different flow characteristics. This may allow the use of smaller needles (Restylane Silk, Belotero, Refyne, Volbella). In some techniques, a less-free-flowing filler may be chosen if very small amounts of filler are desirable and injections need to be more controlled.

Different HA products tend to have different degrees of hydrophilicity. In areas where more precise injections are desirable (white roll of the lip, tear trough) a less hydrophilic product (Restylane, Refyne, Volbella, Belotero) may be desired as opposed to areas where a more "pillowy" effect is desired (cheek mound, body of the lip) where perhaps a more hydrophilic product would be preferred (Juvederm).

G-prime, or elastic modulus, is a much talked about feature of HA fillers. In general terms, the higher the G-prime, the more cohesive the product and theoretically the more "lifting potential" the product has. The lower the G-prime, the softer the product, the more likely it is to flatten or spread and the "less supportive" the product. If, for example more "lift" is desired as in the cheek mound, a high G-prime product is desirable (Voluma, Restylane Lyft). Intermediate G-prime products have the widest range of applications as they provide some "lift" and some "fill." The lowest G-prime products produce mostly "fill" with little to no lift due to their easy deformation and less cohesiveness. (Restylane Silk, Juvederm Ultra, Belotero) This is a very general classification and only with experience can a practitioner choose the best filler for a particular application.

In choosing the appropriate filler, several variables should be considered:

1) Depth of the line or groove to be filled.
    a) Fine lines such as radial perioral lines are best addressed with the thinner, lower viscosity fillers (Restylane Silk, Refyne, Juvederm Ultra, Volbella, or

Belotero). These can very carefully be used in the glabellar furrows in those that do not respond completely to neurotoxin treatment.

b) Intermediate depth lines such as shallow labiomandibular or melolabial grooves or circumoral lines are best treated with medium thickness Hyaluronic acid fillers (Restylane, Defyne, Juvederm Ultra Plus, Vollure).

c) Deeper grooves can be addressed with the densest fillers such as Restylane Lyft or Radiesse.

2) Proposed depth of injection

a) If injections will be at the mid or deep dermal level or just subdermal, caution should be exercised to not use too dense a material or a material that is not well suited for intradermal injection.

b) Even the least dense HA fillers should be used carefully as too superficial an injection can result in nodules.

c) Injected too superficially, HA fillers can result in a Tyndall effect. This results from a scattering of light from the particles of hyaluronic acid that are suspended in a colloidal gel. The net result is a blue hue that can be quite visible, particularly in areas of thin skin such as the naso-jugal groove.

d) Pre-periosteal injections, as in cheek mound enhancement, can be performed with any product. Here denser products tend to create a more significant correction. Voluma, Radiesse, and Restylane Lyft are the volumizers of choice. Although a relatively "safer" plane of injection with less incidence of nodularity and Tyndall effect, caution should be exercised to avoid excessive bruising and equal care should be taken in avoiding intravascular injection of any of the products.

e) In treating deeply, with the objective of increasing midfacial volume, 5 poly-L-lactic acid is a great choice for stimulating collagen production wherever fibroblasts are found [13]. As such, injection of 5-poly-L-lactic acid in a number of tissue layers can stimulate collagen synthesis and results in an "expansion" of the treated tissues. Of note is the fact that the results with Sculptra are not immediate (four to six weeks until final results are seen) and may require multiple treatment sessions.

f) Polymethylmethacrylate, by virtue of its permanence, should be reserved for deeper injection, subdermal or pre-periosteal. Recent approval for more superficial injection for acne scars has been given, however, this author has little experience with this technique. Overcorrection should be avoided when using polymethylmethacrylate. Patients should be allergy test to bovine collagen as the material is suspended in a bovine collagen gel.

3) Thickness of skin in the area being treated

a) Injection into very thin skin with any product other than the thinnest viscosity HA fillers is not recommended.

b) Areas with thicker skin are more forgiving and can accept treatment with most of the intermediate viscosity fillers and some of the denser fillers as well.

c) Radiesse, due to its dense viscosity, paste like consistency and opacity, should be reserved for subdermal treatment only in areas of intermediate to thick skin.

d) Poly-L-lactic acid can be injected from subdermis down to periosteum, however, more superficial injections do raise the risk of nodule formation. Using a more dilute preparation of the product, distributing the product at the time of injection, massaging the area directly after injection and instructing patient to massage several times a day for several days helps mitigate the chance of nodule formation [14].

   e) Polymethylmethacrylate, as mentioned earlier, should only be used in areas of thick skin
4) How much volume is desired
   a) If the target of treatment is effacing specific lines, the various HA fillers are the best choices. Calcium hydroxylapatite and polymethylmethacrylate can also be considered.

   b) If the aim of treatment is global volume replacement, the densest HA fillers (Restylane Lyft, Voluma) or collagen inducers (Sculptra, Radiesse) should be used.

6.8 Technical Pearls

Various techniques of injection have been recommended (Figure 6.14). Linear threading is the most commonly used technique to place filler along the axis of a line or groove. With anterograde linear threading, product is deposited as the

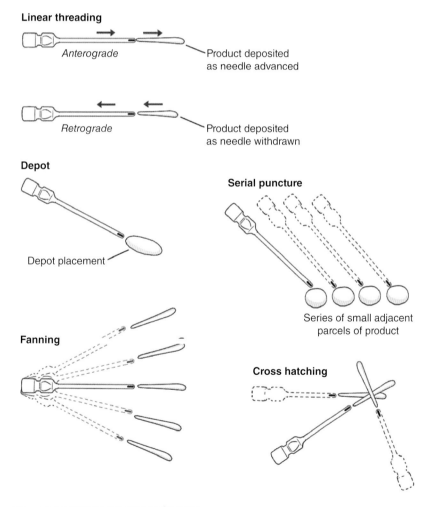

Figure 6.14 Various injection techniques.

needle or cannula is advanced. In the retrograde technique, the needle is advanced without depositing product and as the needle or cannula is backed out, filler is deposited. With the exception of the vermilion border where anterograde injection is used, it is this author's preference to inject in retrograde fashion. This recommendation is based on the increased safety in avoiding intravascular injection using a retrograde technique.

Depot technique involves placing parcels of product at a desired depth. This technique is useful in raising depressed scars or in placing deep depot injections in cheek mounds or temporal hollows.

Serial puncture is placement of very small depot injections along a line or fold. The benefit is the ability to accurately place the desired volume at different points along a line. The disadvantage is the potential for discontinuous "beads" of product that can be palpable or visible. Additionally, given the larger number of injections sites, the risk of bruising may be higher. Advocates of this technique feel there may a lesser chance of entering a vessel if the needle is not being passed through longer distances in a subdermal plane.

Fanning and cross hatching involve entering the skin and depositing product in a fan shaped or cross hatched fashion. This results in a "lattice-like" pattern in areas requiring more diffuse volume enhancement. This technique is particularly useful when using poly-L-lactic acid with injections placed diffusely into multiple planes.

6.9   Needles vs. Cannulas

This topic is the source of much debate with advocates on both sides. Those who recommend cannulas cite the increased safety suggesting less incidence of soft tissue trauma, bruising, and intravascular injection. Those who have used needles all along will note that by penetrating tissue more sharply, there is less tissue trauma, less bruising, and no significant difference between sharp needles and blunt cannulas in the incidence of vascular penetration and intravascular injection.

From this author's perspective, having been referred equal numbers of patients, with equal severity of injury from intravascular injection, from both cannula- and needle-treated groups, the decision on which to use should be based on operator confidence and facility.

One distinct advantage of needle use is the ability to inject material into any desired tissue layer. Mid or deep reticular dermis, dermal/subdermal junction, deep subdermal, supraperiosteal, and even sub periosteal planes are accessible with sharp needle injection. Cannulas will tend to find a path of least resistance and make targeting a specific skin or soft tissue layer somewhat more challenging. Blunt instruments also tend to have more tissue drag (as may be seen in the use of a taper suture needle vs a cutting needle when suturing) and this may lead to more soft tissue trauma on injection. Lastly, cannulas tend to give a false sense of confidence and may make the injector less vigilant in their injection technique.

6.10   Specific Injection Pearls

6.10.1   Fine Lines

Preferred products for fine line injection are Restylane Silk, Restylane Refyne, Volbella, and Belotero. The preferred technique is retrograde linear threading although some practitioners recommend fanning or cross hatching oblique to the axis of the lines. Be careful to inject at or below the deep reticular dermis to avoid nodules or Tyndall effect.

6.10.2   Melolabial Groove

Preferred products are Restylane, Restylane Lyft, Restylane Defyne, Juvederm Ultra Plus, Vollure, Radiesse. Preferred technique

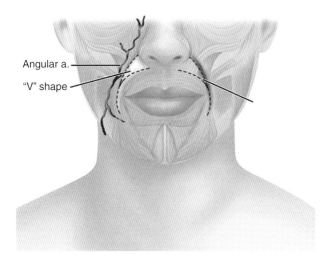

Angular a.

"V" shape

Figure 6.15 Staying medial to the groove will yield the best results. A "V" shaped injection in a fan-like fashion superiorly will help fill the depression at the alar groove.

is retrograde linear threading injecting along the depth of the groove from lateral to medial. Key point here is always to err on the side of injecting slightly medial to the groove. Injection lateral to the groove, or migration of product lateral to the groove with zygomatic contraction and smiling, can lead to exaggeration of the groove by making the fold of tissue lateral to the groove heavier (Figure 6.15).

Placement of filler in a "V" shaped pattern at the superior portion of the groove as one approaches the alar groove can result in a significant improvement. Extreme caution should be exercised in this anatomic "triangle" to avoid intravascular injection into branches of the angular artery.

6.10.3   Labiomandibular Groove

Similar recommendations regarding product and injection technique. Again, err on the side of injecting more medially to avoid making the fold of tissue lateral to the labimandibular groove heavier. Injection at the superior end of this groove, at the lateral commissure, can create an illusion of elevation of the corners of the mouth and reduction of

the "marionette-like" posturing of the lateral lip (Figure 6.16).

Care should be taken to avoid branches of the facial artery, specifically the inferior labial branch. Bruising in this area is common due to the superficially coursing inferior labial vein.

6.10.4   Pre Jowl Sulcus

At the inferior-most aspect of the labiomandibular groove lies the pre jowl sulcus. Injection of relatively denser materials (Restylane Lyft, Radiesse, Juvederm Ultra Plus) in a supraperiosteal plane can be effective in softening the scalloped appearance of the jawline. As previously described, injection should always be biased medially so as not to make the jowl itself heavier (Figure 6.17).

The same vascular system is at risk as described in labiomandibular goove injections.

6.10.5   Labiomental Groove

Low or intermediate viscosity hyaluronic acid fillers are preferred in treating the labiomental groove. The dermis is more adherent at the depth of the groove and

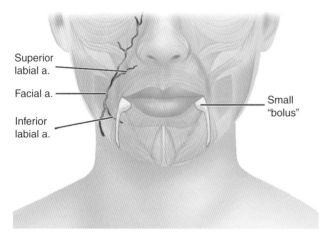

Figure 6.16 A small bolus of material placed right below the lateral commissure will help elevate the corners of the mouth.

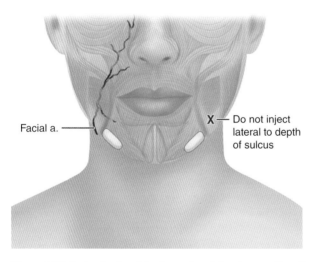

Figure 6.17 Pre jowl sulcus injections placed deeply can efface the scalloped appearance of the jawline creating a smoother contour.

injections are somewhat more painful. Too superficial of an injection can result in nodules that may have a blue hue. Patients should be advised that post injection erythema may persist longer here than in other areas of the face (Figure 6.18).

6.10.6 Midface Volumization

In many case of deep melolabial grooves, a contributing component is loss or redistribution of midfacial soft tissue volume with resultant loss of midfacial support. As such, patients who are volume deficient in this area are good candidates for volume replacement. Historically, this was achieved by placement of cheek implants. Transfer of fat has been, and continues to be, a popular technique to replace or augment midfacial volume.

Several excellent products have been developed to volumize the midface. Voluma, Restylane Lyft, and Radiesse are effective in creating improvement in the

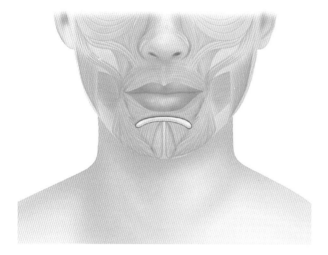

Figure 6.18 Labiomental groove injections can decrease the appearance of a deep sulcus.

midface contour. Injections are generally performed in a depot fashion in a deep, supraperiosteal plane. Injections here should be placed inferior to the attachment of the orbital septum onto the inferior orbital rim. Placement of a finger along the inferior orbital rim can guide injections away from the lower eyelid (Figure 6.19a).

Prior to injections, the desired areas of augmentation are marked on the patient. The pattern of injection often resembles the crescentic shape of a cheek implant. The thought of "non-surgical" cheek augmentation is appealing to most patients. Bruising can occur if any deep or superficial vessels are violated. Perpendicular placement of the needle or cannula down to the supraperiosteal plane is preferred to entering tangentially and passing through a longer distance to reach the injection site. By traversing less tissue with a needle or cannula, bruising can be minimized.

Poly-L-lactic acid is another good option for midface volumization. Unlike HA or calcium hydroxylapatite fillers, which show an immediate result, Sculptra requires induction of collagen and may require four to six weeks for results to become visible

[14]. Generally two to three sessions may be required with some patients with significant volume deficiencies requiring additional sessions (Figure 6.19b).

Pearls for Sculptra include:

1) Reconstitute product at least 48 hours prior to use.
2) Use a dilute concentration of the product (5 cc sterile water for initial reconstitution, 3–5 additional ccs sterile water and 0.5–1 cc of 1% lidocaine with epinephrine added prior to injection) to avoid clogging of needles and a more uniform distribution of product.
3) Keep the diluted solution in a bath of warm water during injection.
4) Use a 3 cc luer lock syringe
5) Use a 25 gauge 1″ needle that should be changed frequently to avoid clogging.
6) Inject the material in several planes to achieve diffuse stimulation of fibroplasts and collagen production
7) Massage the injected area to distibute the product more uniformly. This is best done right after the injections taking advantage of the lidocaine effect.
8) Have patients self-massage for a 5x a day for five days to minimize the risk of nodules.

(a)

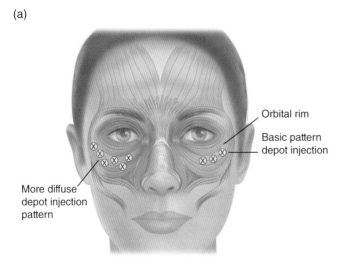

Orbital rim

Basic pattern depot injection

More diffuse depot injection pattern

(b)

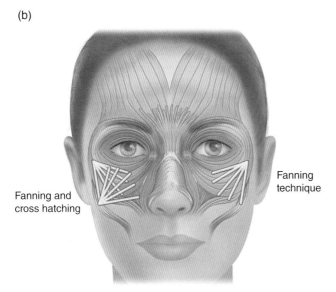

Fanning technique

Fanning and cross hatching

Figure 6.19 (a) Depot injections into the cheek mound after mapping out areas of deficiency can be effective in softening the appearance of melolabial grooves and restoring a "V" shape to the face. (b) Sculptra is injected diffusely into the cheek at various tissue depths to stimulate collagen production and result in "expansion" of cheek volume.

6.10.7 Temporal Hollows

Dense HA fillers (Restylane Lyft, Juvederm Ulra Plus) and poly-L-lactic acid are options for use in temporal hollows. With HA, In order to distribute the volume of material diffusely, some practitioners advocate diluting the product prior to injection. With either type of product, injection should be deep just above the periosteum. Injection should be in a depot fashion for HA and in a diffuse injection fashion for Sculptra.

With both products, generous massage of the area is helpful in avoiding nodules. Significant volumes of HA are generally required and two to three sessions of injection with Sculptra are the norm. As such, the cost/benefit ratio should be reviewed with the patient and unless the hollowing is creating significant facial disharmony, often this anatomic deficiency can be left untreated.

6.10.8   Lips

Lip injections can be one of the most appearance enhancing techniques in facial filler use. Excessive or asymmetric injections, disregard for the ideal ratio of upper lip to lower lip, or poor knowledge of lip anatomy can lead to visibly unnatural results.

Lips should be analyzed for deficiency in definition, vertical height, volume or combinations of these. Most often, the ledge-like "lip" of the vermilion cutaneous junction is lost with age. The cutaneous lip lengthens and the pink lip rolls under effacing the junction between the two and giving the appearance of shorter pink lip height and loss of lip volume.

Restoration of the definition of this vermilion cutaneous junction redefines the contour of the lip and creates the illusion of increased height and volume without affecting projection of the lip or creating amorphous volumization. Generally injection is begun laterally and works toward the ipsilateral peak of cupid's bow. Rarely is the depth of cupid's bow injected as this creates a convexity of this naturally concave contour and looks unnatural.

If the junction of the white and pink lip is augmented, the upper lip may "stand away" from the philtral complex suggesting that the lips were injected. To create better harmony between the lip and the philtral columns, and to enhance the depth of the philtral dimple, small volumes of filler are injected to enhance the philtral columns and improve the continuity of the philtral columns with the augmented white line margin (Figure 6.20a).

If true volume deficiency persists despite the technique described above,

small volumes of filler can be injected directly into the body of the lips where the deficiencies exist. Care should be taken not to overfill the body of the lip, nor create a continuous "sausage like" fullness which lacks definition.

In enhancing the lips, the golden ratio of 1 : 1.6 should be respected. If the upper lip is treated as unity or "1" the lower lip should be 1.6 the size or vertical height of the upper lip (Figure 6.20b). Unattractively augmented lips often will have the upper and lower lips equal in size or in extreme cases, the upper lip bigger than the lower.

Lastly, dental occlusal relationships should be considered in examination of the lips and consideration for treatment. Patients with class II malocclusion, or even subtle posturing of the upper lip anterior to the lower lip, may not be good candidates for upper lip augmentation that may exaggerate the disharmony.

6.10.9   Nasojugal Groove

An abnormally deep nasojugal groove can lead to dark shadowing in the lower lids. In many cases this is accentuated by significant pseudo herniation of lower lid fat and may only benefit from lower eyelid blepharoplasty surgery. In cases without significant fat pseudo herniation or, in patients who are not inclined to consider surgery, judicious injection of HA fillers into the depth of the trough can lessen the shadow effect [15].

Low density, least hydrophilic HA fillers should be used. Restylane, Restylane Silk and Belotero are the main products used in the tear trough.

Injection should be placed deeply just above the periosteum (Figure 6.21) to minimize the chances of Tyndall effect or visibility of the product in this area with extremely thin skin. Despite the best efforts of the injector, a subtle blue hue is not uncommon after injection. Belotero has a slight advantage as there is less

(a)

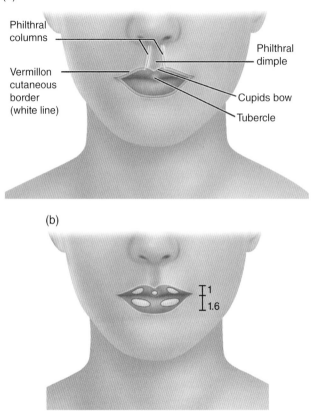

Philthral columns

Philthral dimple

Vermillon cutaneous border (white line)

Cupids bow

Tubercle

(b)

1
1.6

Figure 6.20 (a) Injection along the vermilion/cutaneous border will help restore the "lip" that anatomically is present in youth. Not injecting the concavity of Cupid's bow maintains a natural contour and avoids the "rounded" or "linear" appearance seen in a poorly injected lip. Injecting small volumes along the philtral columns maintains continuity with lip margins and deepens the philtral dimple. (b) The golden ratio of 1 : 1.6 should be respected.

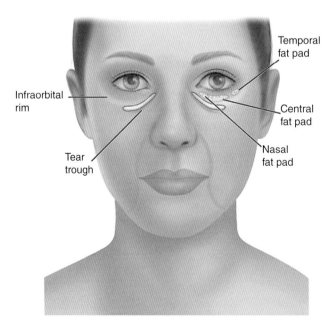

Temporal fat pad

Infraorbital rim

Central fat pad

Nasal fat pad

Tear trough

Figure 6.21 Tear trough injections are placed deeply just above the infraorbital rim periosteum. Minimal volumes of the least hydrophilic product available is recommended to avoid excess fullness or Tyndall effect.

chance of Tyndall effect because of the uniformity of size of the HA particles.

Under injection is advised as all the materials have some degree of hydrophilicity and creating a mound of material often looks worse than the pre-existing concavity.

As this area is highly vascular, bruising is not uncommon.

6.11 Complications of Facial Fillers

6.11.1 Bruising

Bruising is fairly common in the use of fillers. As the dermis and subdermis is invested with a rich plexus of vessels and the target injection plane for many types of filler is the deep dermis or dermal/subdermal junction, bruising is difficult to avoid in every case. Patients should be advised that bruising may occur. All patients are asked if they have any important events within two to three days of their scheduled injection appointment. If so, they are offered the option to come back at a more opportune time.

Bruising can be particularly problematic near the eyes because of the rich vascular plexus and the thinness of the skin (Figure 6.22).

6.11.2 Nodules

Nodules can be seen immediately at the time of injection, or appear several days after the initial swelling associated with injection subsides. If present at the time of injection, gentle massage with redistribution of filler may be all that is necessary. Patients are advised to look at the injected area three to four days post injection. If any small lumps or nodules are visible, gentle massage can flatten these within the first 10 days post injection. Patient are also told that if the nodules are "palpable" but not "visible" they should be left alone so as not to redistribute product away

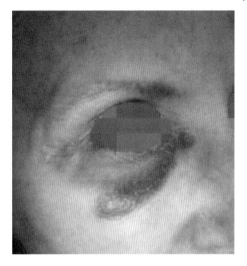

Figure 6.22 Bruising around the eyes is not uncommon as seen in this patient injected in the nasojugal groove.

from the intended injection site or hasten the dissolution of product.

If any visible nodules persist, within two weeks of injection, a small needle puncture (25–20 gauge needle) may allow expression of some of the material. If not possible or if the patient presents later than two weeks, hyaluronidase can be injected to dissolve the material. Initially 5–10 units can be used based on the amount of volume requiring dissolution. (Hylenex is supplied as 15 units per cc, Vitrase as 20 units per cc.) It is best to undertreat with hyaluronidase and retreat as necessary to avoid dissolving too much product and losing the desired correction.

As hyaluronidase is a component of bee venom, patients with sensitivity to bee stings should be advised they may have a brisk erythematous reaction to hyaluronidase injection. Any patient who has severe bee sting allergies should be allergy tested prior to the use of hyaluronidase.

6.11.3 Overcorrection

Overcorrection can be treated with hyaluronidase in the same manner as treating isolated nodules. Here a more dilute solution of hyaluronidase can be injected more diffusely. 10–30 units are injected initially. Diluting 1:1 to 1:3 with saline gives more volume to inject over a larger area than with an isolated nodule

6.11.4 Tyndall Effect

As previously described, placement of HA products too superficially, in too large a volume or in areas of very this skin can cause a Tyndall effect by scattering of light by the particles of HA suspended in the product. Treatment involves dissolution of product with hyaluronidase.

6.11.5 Calcium Hydroxylapatite

Nodules or overcorrection with Radiesse is much more difficult to treat. Initial management is massage of the affected area to try to fragment the bolus of material and stimulate phagocytosis of the particulate matter. Injection of saline into the mass of material may help by breaking up larger masses of material.

In nodules or masses of material that do not adequately respond to this conservative treatment, surgical excision may be required (Figure 6.23).

6.11.6 Sculptra

Nodules or overcorrection with Sculptra can be problematic. When first introduced,

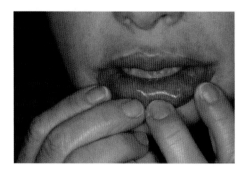

Figure 6.23 Subcutaneous nodules of Radiesse injected into the lip. This required excision of material by resection of mucosa and muscle along the gingivolabial sulcus.

the incidence of nodules was not insignificant and many practitioners avoided using the product based on this. With modification of dilution and injection techniques and with protocols for post-injection massage, the risk of nodules has been negligible.

Dilution and injection pearls have been discussed earlier in this chapter. The importance of placing small aliquots of material in multiple planes of the facial soft tissue is the key to avoiding complications. Being certain injections are not placed too superficially and definitive post-injection massage, initially by the injector and for several days after injection by the patient are equally important.

Avoiding injection into areas with significant muscle activity (e.g. perioral) may also limit nodule formation as there is less chance muscle movement will cause a "mounding" effect of material.

Should nodules occur, massage, and/or intranodule injection with saline or dilute kenalog 10 can be attempted. In recalcitrant cases, surgical excision may be required.

6.11.7 Granuloma Formation

Granulomatous reactions can occur in response to any injectable material and generally occur weeks to months after treatment. Treatment is with intralesional kenalog 10 injections with use of oral steroids in more severe cases. Rarely, surgical excision may be required (Figure 6.24).

6.11.8 Vascular Compromise

No complication of an aesthetic facial filler treatment is more disturbing than vascular compromise. The etiology is thought to be related to extravascular compression of vessels by product or, more likely, intravascular injection of product. Based on the network of vessels affected, this can lead to temporary ischemia of a given distribution to more

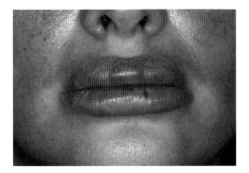

Figure 6.24 Delayed granuloma formation to polyacrylamide gel requiring surgical excision.

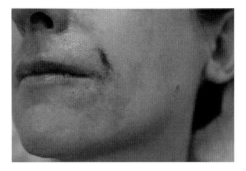

Figure 6.25 Patient was injected into proximal melolabial groove with angiosomal mottling occurring post injection consistent with vascular compromise. Notice distribution along branches of the angular artery including the inferior and superior labial artery branches.

severe ischemia with tissue necrosis. If in the distribution of the ophthalmic artery, end vessel involvement of the retinal artery can lead to blindness. As there are anastomoses between branches of the external carotid (supratrochlear, supraorbital, angular, nasal dorsal a.) and the internal carotid (vessels within the orbit), any intravascular injection in the face can lead to retinal artery occlusion and blindness. Fortunately the complication of blindness is extremely rare. Cutaneous vascular compromise is not as rare and anyone injecting fillers in the face should be aware of the signs and symptoms and be prepared to treat immediately.

Any distortion of vision during injection, any significant cutaneous blanching that does not resolve within seconds, any mottling of the skin at or near the injection site or in a distant angiosomal distribution should be considered a vascular compromise event. Injection should be stopped immediately and an emergency protocol should be initiated (Figure 6.25).

Vascular Compromise Treatment Protocol

1) Stop injection.
2) Apply warm compresses.
3) Massage vigorously.
4) Have the patient CHEW a 325 mg tablet of aspirin. Continue aspirin 650 mg PO daily until vascular compromise resolved

5) Inject hyaluronidase
   a) A minimum of 150 units
   b) Dilute hyaluronidase 4:1 with plain lidocaine (no epi)
   c) Further dilute with saline if more injection volume needed
   d) Inject diffusely in the distribution of proposed ischemia, not necessarily at the injection site of the filler
   e) Reinject in an hour
   f) It is prudent to have six or more vials of hyaluronidase on hand at all times if you plan to inject HA fillers
6) Follow patient for any signs of improvement in ischemia post hyaluronidase
7) Administer Viagra (50 mg sildenafil citrate) assuming patient is not on nitrates. Continue 50 mg daily until process resolved
8) If process is progressive and not responding to above treatments, consider hyperbaric oxygen (HBO) therapy. It is prudent to investigate hyperbaric oxygen availability in your area and protocols for prescribing HBO before an event occurs

The use of nitropaste is controversial. Some advocate the vasodilitory effects while others feel vasodilation may cause propagation of product to more distal end vessels with less chance of successfully dissolving the product within the proximal site of occlusion.

Any skin breakdown is treated with standard skin care protocols as with second or third degree burn injuries. Full thickness necrosis should be debrided as needed. Upon complete healing, "V" beam laser or intense pulsed light (IPL) treatments can be offered to address any persistent erythem or dyspigmentation. If scarring is deeper, excision of the scar with reconstruction may be required.

References

1 Fagien, S. (1999). Botox for the treatment of dynamic and hyperkinetic facial lines and furrows: adjunctive use in facial aesthetic surgery. *Plast. Reconstr. Surg.* 103: 701–708.

2 Ahn, M.S., Catten, M., and Maas, C.S. (2000). Temporal brow lift using botulinum toxin A. *Plast. Reconstr. Surg.* 105: 1129–1135.

3 Alam, M., Dover, J.S., Klein, A.W. et al. (2002). Botulinum A exotoxin for hyperfunctional facial lines: where not to inject. *Arch. Dermatol.* 138: 1180–1185.

4 Brandt, F.S. and Boker, A. (2003). Botulinum toxin for rejuvenation of the neck. *Clin. Dermatol.* 21: 513–520.

5 Carruthers, J.A., Lowe, N.J., Menter, M.A. et al. (2002). A multicenter, double-blind, randomized, placebo-controlled study of efficacy and safety of botulinum toxin type A in the treatment of glabellar lines. *J. Am. Acad. Dermatol.* 46: 840–849.

6 Donath, A.S., Glasgold, R.A., Meier, J. et al. (2010). Quantitative evaluation of volume augmentation in the tear trough with a hyaluronic acid based filler: a three dimensional analysis. *Plast. Reconstr. Surg.* 125: 1515–1522.

7 Jones, D. and Vleggaar, D. (2007). Technique for injecting poly-L-lactic acid. *J. Drugs Dermatol.* 6: S13–S17.

8 Klein, A. (2003). Botulinum toxin complications. *Dermatol. Surg.* 29: 549–556.

9 Larrabee, W.F. and Makielski, K.H. (1993). *Surgical Anatomy of the Face*, 49–59. New York: Raven Press.

10 Matarasso, S.L. and Matarasso, A. (2001). Treatment guidelines for botulinum toxin type A for the periocular region and a report on partial upper lip ptosis following injections to the lateral canthal rhytids. *Plast. Reconstr. Surg.* 108: 208–214.

11 Park, J., Hoagland, T., and Park, M. (2003). Anatomy of the corrugator supercilii muscle. *Arch. Facial Plast. Surg.* 5: 412–415.

12 Rohrich, R. and Pessa, J. (2007). The fat components of the face: anatomy and clinical implications for cosmetic surgery. *Plast. Reconstr. Surg.* 119: 2219–2227.

13 Vleggaar, D. and Bauer, U. (2004). Facial enhancement and the European experience with Sculptra. *J. Drugs Dermatol.* 3: 542–547.

14 Wise, J.B. and Greco, T. (2006). Injectable treatments for the aging face. *Facial Plast. Surg.* 22: 140–146.

15 Wu, W.T. (2010). Botox facial slimming/facial sculpting: the role of botulinum toxin-A in the treatment of hypertrophic massetereic muscle and parotid enlargement to narrow the lower facial width. *Facial Plast. Surg. Clin. North Am.* 18: 133–140.

7

Building Your Practice

Jay R. Levine

PBHS Inc., Santa Rosa, CA, USA

Practice growth can be achieved in many ways, but one thing is certain: successful practices consistently allocate time and resources to a marketing strategy. They pay close attention to how they are perceived in their community *and* online and are proactive about protecting their reputation.

Practice marketing takes on many forms. While traditional styles such as postcards, mailers, and print ads are still important, the modern practice knows that its online presence should not be ignored, as the Internet presents a wonderful chance to connect with potential patients in the area.

7.1 Internet Marketing: *What's in it for you?*

People no longer check the phone book when looking for health providers – they are more likely to "go online" to search for and evaluate potential professionals in the area. A search on Google will quickly deliver the business listings and practice websites of providers in the area … *is yours on the list?*

In Bright Local's annual *Local Consumer Review Survey*, healthcare providers were second only to restaurants in terms of how important reputation is to online users when making a choice [1].

7.2 Promoting Your Practice: Formulating a Strategy

Before embarking on any marketing journey, it's best to have a clear idea of what you want to get out of it. What are your goals and expected outcomes? Are you looking to attract new patients or expand reach into a new community? Or are you a busy practice that simply wants to stay in touch, educate, and promote to current patients?

Once you have these goals laid out, you are ready to begin your marketing journey. To get started, decide how much money you will allocate toward marketing. If you aren't sure of what your marketing budget should be – 3–5% for more established practices, and up to 7% for a new practice can be considered.

When determining your marketing budget and researching consultants, keep in mind that even the most basic marketing plans today should incorporate these fundamentals:

- Logo for brand recognition in print and digital materials
- Educational Website promoting services, doctors, and contact information
- Locally targeted online and print marketing campaigns

Neurotoxins and Fillers in Facial Esthetic Surgery, First Edition. Edited by Bradford M. Towne and Pushkar Mehra.
© 2019 John Wiley & Sons, Inc. Published 2019 by John Wiley & Sons, Inc.
Companion website: www.wiley.com/go/towne/neurotoxins

- Up-to-date business listings on online platforms
- Online review monitoring
- Branded social media pages

7.3 Website Design Companies

When choosing providers of these services, keep in mind that *inexpensive* sometimes means *inexperienced*. By contrast, putting your brand in the hands of a highly experienced, professional firm that has focused on *your* specialty in *your* market will likely yield better results than can be expected of a freelance web designer, or a design company that normally works outside your industry. An experienced company will also help to avoid a costly branding mistake that could quickly turn into a public relations (PR) nightmare.

7.4 Building Your Brand

A brand is more than just a logo. It is the feeling people have about you, the experiences they have had with you, and those they expect to have when they walk through your door. It's the relationship you have with your community, including other practices, existing patients, and potential ones. An effective marketing strategy accelerates the branding process through a variety of channels – print, digital, and social media to name a few – and it does so with strict consistency to further enhance recognition.

The first step in building your brand is a great logo. The logo should convey your values and give people a feel for your practice before they have even met you. Look for a reputable graphic designer or agency who understands your specialty and your location. It is the most important visual aspect of your marketing strategy, increasingly so as it becomes recognizable and, hopefully, sharable.

7.5 Print Marketing

With print marketing, it's time to let your brand shine! Printing your logo on stationery, mugs, patient education materials, and signage will help to solidify your brand in the eyes of your community. In addition, mailers such as postcards, coupons, and newsletters are all still great ways to connect with existing patients as a reminder to come in, and new patients as an incentive to schedule an initial appointment.

7.6 Website Design: Choosing a Designer

When selecting a website design firm, you will want to make sure that they have adequate experience in designing websites for *your* specialty. Ask for examples and "test" those websites to see if they rank well on Google and Bing. Does the firm provide adequate, user-friendly information for patients while meeting the search ranking needs of the client? A good website design company should be able to deliver on all of these requirements, and will provide the following benefits to your practice:

- In-depth, up-to-date use of design and technological trends, including search engine algorithms, mobile device access and aesthetic appeal. This knowledge should be applied regularly to your website for optimal performance.
- Content management access. You should be given login information so that you can edit website content as needed.
- Additional services such as secure email, patient registration, and scheduling forms.
- Industry knowledge to provide adequate content and an understanding of your target audience.
- An exquisite, engaging design that will capture the interest of potential patients.

- Data on your audience and website performance.
- Peace of mind. Knowing that this part of your marketing strategy is in the experienced hands of a company with a long history of happy clients eases the burden on a business owner.

7.6.1   Other Items to Consider when Choosing a Website Designer

How Much Input Do You Want to Have? Are you "hands-off" when it comes to marketing, or do you want to be involved at every step, starting with the choosing of basic design elements?

Pricing: While it is always tempting to save money, creating a website that is responsive and ranks well in searches is not a "Do it yourself (DIY)" job for most people. It takes industry-knowledge, experience, a thoughtful approach and time. Would your time be better spent seeing more patients or with your family? Often what seems like a good deal ends in a low-quality website that cannot rank well by Google due poor technical design.

Website Content: Don't forget about website content – the words that explain your services and methodologies and convey a sense of your "practice personality." Without content, prospective patients (and search engines) will simply pass you by and look for information elsewhere. You have a few options when it comes to website content. Some designers offer fully custom content (the priciest option) or stock content (less expensive) that you can customize yourself. A third option is a website without any content at all. *Be careful not to take content from elsewhere on the Internet, as this will quickly get you in trouble for copyright infringement.*

When comparing prices between website designers, make sure to factor in the cost of content that you will need.

A user-friendly *and* search-engine-friendly website includes:

- A home page with a great mission statement;
- Doctor and staff bios;
- One page for each service that you offer; and
- Contact and registration information

Keep in mind that a lack of content and "keyword-stuffing" are frowned upon by search engines, and can even result in penalties.

No matter which route you choose for obtaining website content, you will want to make sure to read through it thoroughly before taking the website live to ensure that it accurately represents your practice.

Portfolio: Take a look at the designer's portfolio. Do you like the way the sites look on your desktop? What about on a mobile device? Do a quick search on Google for the key services you provide and your location to see how they rank.

Technicalities: Does your website designer get the technical details right? Very important for patient experience and search engine rankings is the accessibility of your website. Google expects your website to be user friendly, easy for users to navigate and with ample information about the services you offer. A good website designer can balance the needs of patients with the expectations of search engines without the user ever knowing it. Some of the most basic technical elements are:

- Responsive design for various screen sizes
- Phone number links for mobile use
- Contact forms
- Blog functionality
- Meaningful content – avoid "keyword-stuffing"
- Social media and testimonial integration
- Security

Member Associations: A great source for website design and other marketing recommendations is your national professional member association. Who do they endorse?

7.6.2 Designing Your Website

Once you have chosen your website designer, it's time to start building. The following are some tried-and-true concepts to create a practice website that speaks to your audience, to Google *and* to you.

7.6.2.1 Connect with the User

Engage your audience with a clean, modern design that reflects your brand and mission. The design of your website should also take into consideration the demographics of your community. What will speak to them?

Encourage interaction with:

- *Social Media Links:* Encourage social media interaction by placing icons with links to your social media channels near the top of your home page, and on interior pages as well.
- *Local Interest:* Incorporate pictures of local landmarks and stock models whose demographics match those of your town to give potential patients a welcoming feel.
- *Promotions:* If your office has any special offers such as new patient specials, free consultations, and so on add these to your website in a prominent place to attract more patients.
- *Make it Easy to Contact You*: Clickable phone links and a "call to action" statement should head each page so that patients can easily click and call you from their mobile phones.

7.6.2.2 Outside Perspective

Your needs are probably different than those of your patients. For example, a picture that seems interesting to you may be frightening to a patient. *So ask yourself this question:* "If I were a patient, what elements would I want to see (or NOT see) on this website?" Most patients do not want to see or read anything that is too clinical or scary. Blood and needles are generally not advised, as are any other potentially disturbing surgical or otherwise graphic images. *So what should you post?* Before and after pictures (with permission) are great for keeping your audience interested and hopeful about their own treatment options. Office events, industry jokes, and charity information are all fair game as well.

7.6.2.3 Accuracy

The content that you have on your website should accurately reflect the services you offer, the brands that you use, and the details of your policies. Including procedures (or brands) that you don't use in your practice just to catch the attention of potential patients will result in fewer conversions and more meaningless interactions. Focus on what you do to get users to convert.

7.6.2.4 Doctor Bios – How Important Are They?

Did you know that the second most often viewed webpage (after the homepage) on a health provider's website is the biography? The doctor bio is very important to patients – it gives them a sense of your experience and your personality, all in one glance. Simply share your academic background, professional experience, and a few general details of your life such as your favorite sports team, which community you proudly live in, and your hobbies.

7.6.2.5 Accessibility

Ensure easy access to all of the information a patient could possibly want by using categories and menu headers. This will make it obvious where patients can find information on procedures, policies, and doctor information. A built-in bonus of having a well-organized website is that it makes it easier for search engines to index your site.

7.6.2.6 Additional Features

For just a small fee (or free), you should be able to incorporate these add-on functions into the website to make life easier for your patients (and you):

- Patient registration forms (Health Insurance Portability and Accountability Act [HIPAA] Compliant, Secure)
- Contact forms
- Scheduling forms
- Informed consent with online signature ability
- Credit card and other online payment options
- Interactive map for directions
- Secure collaboration with referring doctors
- Testimonials

7.6.3 SEO: More on Search Engines

"SEO" stands for Search Engine Optimization, the process by which website administrators work to raise a website's rank in search results. There are many factors that affect SEO. Some are very technical, requiring a website developer to execute, but there are a few basic steps you can take on your own to get the process started.

7.6.3.1 Five Basic SEO Steps you can Take Yourself

1) Claim your Google listing through Google Maps. If you don't see your address, you can create a listing for yourself. Use Google My Business to optimize your listing. Double check the address and phone number for accuracy and add your website uniform resource locator (URL), hours, and a short bio for users to see.
2) Check other directories such as Bing Places, National Provider Identifier (NPI) Database, Facebook, Superpages, CitySearch, and Yellowpages for NAP (Name, Address, and Phone Number). The listings should be consistent across the board on all directories.

3) Encourage positive reviews. Ask happy patients to leave you reviews on the major review sites such as Google, Yelp, RateMDs, and Healthgrades.
4) Update content regularly (see "Blogging," below). Search engines like to see that a website is being maintained regularly. Keep your website up to date by adding procedures and brands as you include them in your practice, or use your blog as a place to share information about new procedures, offers, or practice news.
5) Keep tabs on your progress with Google Analytics. Because of personalized search results, *Googling* search terms for which you want to rank isn't always the best way to judge your search rankings. A better way is with Google Analytics, a free program that delivers search information about your website to you.

Google Analytics – Basic Features to Monitor

- *Bounce Rate:* A "bounce" refers to someone visiting your site and then leaving right away. It may indicate a user who quickly found something they were looking for such as your phone number, or a user that couldn't find what they were looking for quickly and left. Bounce rates over 60% are considered high and may signal the need for a different design or additional content on the site.
- *Traffic Increase:* Keeping in mind that it takes search engines many months to index and register changes to a website, you should see traffic slowly growing over time.
- *Visitor Location:* Sometimes, traffic may come from outside of your area, or even your state or country. Because you are a local business, that traffic is not useful to you, and may indicate the need for a shift in marketing strategies.
- *Time on Site:* This indicates how engaging your site is. Users should

be staying on your site for at least two minutes, otherwise you may want to look at what need your site is not fulfilling for them.

7.6.3.2 Blogging

Blogging is a popular way for connecting with both patients and referring partners. Regular blogging can help with SEO by providing fresh, relevant content to the site, and it also can be syndicated to social media to increase reach and stir up conversation about your practice or your topic. When blogging, anything goes as long as it is not inappropriate, overly graphic or frightening in its nature, and does not violate HIPAA rules.

7.6.3.3 SEO: When to Call in the Experts

SEO professionals are experts in reading Google Analytics and can troubleshoot search-ranking problems quickly before they turn into disasters. Because of some of the more technical aspects of SEO, it is generally recommended that practices consult with a professional. Here are some scenarios that definitely indicate the need for professional help:

1) Major transitions (moving, having just opened, etc.)
2) Competitive locations
3) Multiple locations
4) Changing website domains
5) New practice name
6) New phone number

7.6.4 Online Ads: PPC with Google AdWords

With pay-per-click (PPC) ads, businesses pay for ad space at the top of search results pages, but are only charged a fee when a user clicks on the ad. On Google, the platform is called *Google AdWords*. PPC can be a good option for those who are starting out in competitive markets, as it may take months or even years to rank well

organically in those areas. Some strong indicators that you may want to run an AdWords campaign are:

- *New Practices:* If you are not ranking well organically in your location after starting a new practice, AdWords may give you the boost that you need to break into the market.
- *Competitive Markets:* If there are 10 or more practices in your area competing for the same search term organically, you may want to consider going after that term with a PPC campaign.
- *Specials:* If you are offering a special or coupon, this is a great way to get the word out.
- *Specific Procedure:* Targeting for a specific procedure, especially one that is not widely available in the area, is a great use of paid ad space.
- *Geo-Targeting:* If you would like to increase your reach into surrounding areas, AdWords allows you to target markets geographically.

7.6.4.1 Managing AdWords

While very basic PPC campaigns can usually be managed adequately by most practices on their own, hiring a professional will yield additional benefits that you may not have the time or the wherewithal to obtain on your own:

- Return on investment (ROI) tracking
- Recorded incoming calls
- A/B testing
- Aggressive campaigns
- Highly competitive areas
- Drip marketing email campaigns to further engage and convert prospective patients

7.6.5 Social Media: Getting Started

As with many things in life, the more you put into social media, the more you will get out of it.

7.6.5.1 The Three Es of Social Marketing

- *Educational:* Users like content that teaches them something about health or how to live a better life. Educational posts are attention grabbing for people of all ages.

- *Engaging:* Social media is supposed to encourage engagement, conversation, and the sharing of ideas between people. Spur engagement with office pictures or ask a question of your audience and let them take it from there.
- *Entertaining:* Everyone loves a good joke or a dose of animal-cuteness from time to time. Tell your favorite industry joke, or post a picture of your puppy visiting the office.

7.6.5.2 How to Gain Followers

The goal of social media is to interact with patients and, hopefully, to gain some new ones. So while it is important to create social media pages for your practice, even if you don't plan on using them often, to fully take advantage of this new style of word-of-mouth marketing you will want to establish a reliable fan base.

Here are some tried and true ways to increase social media fans:

1) *Ask* your friends, family, and staff to follow you. That way, when they share your post, their friends will see it too – this is the "viral" nature of social media.
2) *Raffle* off a prize – patients can enter the raffle by "liking" your Facebook page and notifying you (be sure to follow any applicable rules and regulations when running contests and campaigns).
3) *Charitable campaigns* are a great way to promote a cause that is important to you and engage with your community. They also tend to "go viral" because of their charitable nature. Post a notice on your Facebook page saying that for each new like during a certain month, you will donate $1 to a specific charity or organization.
4) *Link* to your social media pages on your website and in your email signature and encourage colleagues to connect with you online.

7.6.5.3 Facebook

In 2016, 47% of consumers recommended a local business on Facebook [2]. Time and time again, Facebook has asserted itself as the most popular online social network, and it should be the first stop on *your* social media marketing journey. Posting one to three times a week is a great target for a busy practice. However, even if you don't post regularly, you should still create a free Facebook business page and brand it with your logo and basic practice information.

Minimum Facebook Page Elements:

- Cover photo
- Profile picture (this is a great place to use your logo)
- Your practice name
- Location
- Phone number
- Website URL
- Office hours
- Services and mission statement

7.6.5.4 Instagram

A social media app designed for mobile use, Instagram allows users to take pictures or videos and share with other Instagram users and even syndicate to other social platforms such as Facebook. Instagram is, by design, a very visually oriented platform: pictures do better than words. Post (with permission) before and after photos or industry news with a #hashtag for better coverage.

7.6.5.5 Twitter

With over 300 million monthly users [3], Twitter is still a social marketing titan. Because of its emphasis on short and sweet posts (140 characters) and the use of #hashtags, Twitter is a great place to "Tweet" about specials and events and send out last-minute announcements.

7.6.5.6 YouTube

Videos are a very popular media form on the Internet. Patient testimonials are easy to capture with a cell phone camera and a steady hand, as are office-tour videos and doctor introductions. Create a YouTube account and upload to your channel. You can then embed the code on your website and share the link on Facebook to further spread the word.

7.6.5.7 Pinterest

Pinterest is like a digital bulletin board where users can collect pictures, recipes and ideas that interest them. This is a great place to share DIY tips and before and after success stories. Be sure to follow other Pinterest users to keep the conversation going.

7.6.5.8 LinkedIn

LinkedIn is a professional networking site – a great place to connect with colleagues and also a place to list your credentials and services. It can also be used to recruit employees or connect with vendors.

7.7 Protecting Your Practice Online

When posting on social media sites, be very careful to avoid the following items:

- *Copyright Infringement:* Be careful not to post anyone else's content without his or her permission first. It's okay to share *links* to content, but don't use copy and paste features unless you have permission from the creator.
- *HIPAA Violations:* Never post pictures, names, clinical, or other identifying details about patients without their written consent.
- *Graphic Content:* Avoid posting pictures that contain blood, heavy bruising or needles in them, as they can be off-putting or frightening to potential patients.
- *Unprofessional Images:* Posting pictures of your office parties and celebrations is great, just make sure that they show you and your staff in a professional light.

7.8 Internet Marketing: Measuring Your Progress

After a few months of active Internet marketing using the steps listed previously, it's time to assess your progress. Google Analytics will tell you how many people are visiting your website and where they come from, and Facebook insights can show you statistics about your Facebook fans, but *how do you know if Internet marketing is truly converting users into patients?* The answer is simple: Ask them. On your patient registration form, in an appointment follow-up email, anywhere you can, start collecting data on what channels are influencing patients in their decision to visit your office. Unlike the standard "How did you find us?" question on your new patient registration form, expand your approach to be open ended and encourage more thoughtful responses. For example, "Did you visit any of these sources when researching providers? (Check all that apply.)" This is a more engaging and comprehensive question that will give you a better idea whether your website and social media pages are influencing patient choice. If you are concerned about the results you find, it may be time to consider hiring a marketing company who knows your specialty well and understands your local market.

7.9 Marketing Is Communication

By putting your brand out there and supporting it across multiple platforms in both print and digital forms, you are well on your way toward building something exceptional – a healthy practice that serves patients in your neighborhood well, is engaged in community events, and grows progressively over time. And it's the simple act of (marketing) communication that will get you there.

Marketing requires time, creativity, strategy, patience, and follow-through, but it has never been more important, as more and more people turn to the Internet for information on your practice. Don't be left out in the cold – by taking the simple steps listed earlier, and enlisting the help of professionals along the way, your practice will experience significant growth for many years to come.

References

1 "Local Consumer Review Survey 2015." BrightLocal. http://www.brightlocal.com/learn/local-consumer-review-survey-2015.

2 "Local Consumer Review Survey 2016." BrightLocal. http://www.brightlocal.com/learn/local-consumer-review-survey.

3 "Number of monthly active Twitter users worldwide from 1st quarter 2010 to 4th quarter 2016 (in millions)." Statista. https://www.statista.com/statistics/282087/number-of-monthly-active-twitter-users.

Index

a

Abobotulinum toxin A   20, 21, 75, 76
advertising, online   108
age of patients   25
aging   10–13
  at different structural levels   47
  factors in   10–11
  and fat distribution   47–48
  Glogau classification   15
  reversing/masking signs of   13
  in specific facial areas   11–13
  theories of   10
allergic reaction, to BoNTA   22
allogeneic facial fillers   51, 53
American Society for Aesthetic Plastic
    Surgery   13
American Society of Plastic Surgeons   47
Artecol   53
Autologen   51, 54, 56, 57
autologous facial fillers   48, 51. *See also*
    specific fillers

b

Belotero   64, 67, 92, 97
biodegradable facial fillers   51, 52, 59
blogging   108
blood supply to face   10
Botox Cosmetic   20–22, 26–28, 30, 76
botulinum neurotoxin A (BoNTA)   19–43
  clinical usage   24–41
  contraindications to treatment   23–24
  diffusion   22–23, 88
  dosing   22

duration of action   22–23
  facial asymmetries secondary to muscle
      paralysis   51
  manufacturing process   20, 22–24
  physiology and characteristics   20, 21
  post-treatment recommendations and
      complications   41–43
  storage and preparation   26–28
botulinum neurotoxins (BoNTs)   19–21
  medical uses of   19–20
  physiology and characteristics   20, 21
  See also botulinum neurotoxin A
      (BoNTA)
bovine collagen   49, 52, 53, 55, 60, 63
brand building   103
brow asymmetry   35–36
brow descent   11, 12
brow drop   32
browlift, indirect   35
brow ptosis   80, 81, 87
buccal fat pad   8
building your practice   103–111
  brand building   103
  Internet marketing   103, 110
  marketing as communication
      110–111
  online ads   108
  print marketing   104
  promotion strategy   103–104
  social media marketing   108–110
  social media protections   110
  website design   104–108
bunny lines   6, 36, 83

Neurotoxins and Fillers in Facial Esthetic Surgery, First Edition. Edited by Bradford M. Towne
and Pushkar Mehra.
© 2019 John Wiley & Sons, Inc. Published 2019 by John Wiley & Sons, Inc.
Companion website: www.wiley.com/go/towne/neurotoxins

c

calcium hydroxylapatite (CaHA)   50–53,
    71–74
    adverse reactions to   72
    benefits of   57, 58
    brand names and indications   52
    classification of   78
    clinical results of   72
    complications   61
    injection of   55
    medical uses of   71
    nodules or overcorrection with   100
    treatment in practice   72–74
cannulas   65, 73, 92
cheek
    deep medial fat of   8
    facial fasciae and   4
    subcutaneous fat of   2, 3
chin, aging and   12
chin dimpling   37–38, 85, 86
clinical usage of BoNTA   24–41
    age of patient   25
    brow asymmetry correction   35–36
    bunny lines   36
    chin dimpling   37–38
    crow's feet   32, 34–35
    downward-turned commissures of
        mouth   38–39
    forehead   32–34
    general injection tips   28–30
    glabella   30–32
    indirect browlift   35
    lip lengthening   39
    patient consultation   24–25
    patient preparation   28–30
    perioral modifications   36–39
    platysmal bands treatment   39–41
    provider regulations   25–26
    storage and preparation   26–28
    upper face treatment   30–36
    vertical lip lines   36, 37
Clostridium botulinum   19
collagen
    bovine   49, 52, 53, 55, 60, 63
    and calcium hydroxylapatite injections   71
    human   52
    in perioral, nasal, and eyebrow regions   2
    porcine   49, 52, 53
    SMAS and   4

collagen inducers   78
complications
    with BoNTA   34, 36, 41–43
    with calcium hydroxylapatite   61
    with fillers   58–61, 68, 99–102
    with neurotoxins   87–88
contraindications, to BoNTA   23–24
corrugators supercilii muscle   5–7
cosmetic procedures   13–14, 47
cross hatching   91, 92
crow's feet   32, 34–35

d

deep cervical fascia   5
deep fascia/periosteum   1
deep fat compartments   7–8
depot technique   91, 92
depressor anguli oris (DAO)   6, 7, 83, 84
depressor labii inferioris   6, 7
depressor septi muscle   6, 7
depressor supercilii muscle   5–7
dermis   1–2, 11
dextran beads in hyaluronic acid   50, 52
diagram, facial   15, 16
diffusion, of neurotoxins   22–23, 88
dilution, of neurotoxins   27, 75–76
doctor bios, on website   106
dosing, for BoNTA   22
downward-turned commissures of
    mouth   38–39
duration of action (BoNTA)   23
Dysport   20–22, 27–28, 30, 76

e

elastic fibers, SMAS and   4
epidermis   1, 11
expanded polytetrafluoroethylene (e-
    PTFE)   53, 54, 60–61
eyelids   12, 32

f

Facebook   109
facial anatomy   1–10
    deep facial fat compartments   7–8
    fasciae   3–5
    ligamentous structures   8–10
    mimetic muscles   4–7
    skin   1–2
    superficial fat compartments   2–3

facial asymmetries
  brow asymmetry correction   35–36
  documenting preexisting
    asymmetries   15
  secondary to muscle paralysis   51
facial nerve   5, 7
fanning   91, 92
fasciae   1, 3–5, 10
fat atrophy   47–48
fat compartments   2–3, 7–8
fat grafts/injections   48, 52, 54, 56–57,
    59–60
fillers   47–61
  allogeneic   51, 53
  autologous   48, 51
  benefits of   55–58
  biodegradable   51, 52
  calcium hydroxylapatite   71–74
  choosing   89–91
  classifications   51–53, 89
  complications with   58–61, 99–102
  ease of use   53–55
  history of   47–48
  hyaluronic acid   63–69
  injection techniques   91–99
  needles vs. cannulas for   92
  non-autologous   48–51
  nonbiodegradable   53, 54
  off-label use of   51
  synthetic   53
  wisdom in use of   75, 88–89
  xenograft   53
  See also specific fillers
fine line injection   92
Food and Drug Administration (FDA)
    51, 64, 71
forehead
  ligamentous structures   9
  neurotoxin injections for   32–34, 80–81
  subcutaneous fat of   3
  zone of fixation in   9
frontal facial diagram   15, 16
frontalis muscle   5, 7, 25

g

galeal deep fat pad   8
galeal fascia   4–5
glabella   30–32, 67–68, 78–80
glabellar muscles   5–6

Glogau classification   15
Google AdWords   108
G-prime products   89
granuloma formation   100, 101

h

hyaluronic acid (HA)   50, 52, 53, 63–64
hyaluronic acid (HA) fillers   50, 55, 63–69
  available products   64
  benefits of   57, 58
  classification of   78
  clinical indications   64
  complications   60
  downward-turned commissures of
    mouth   38
  glabella   67–68
  injection techniques   64–65
  lips   66, 67
  local anesthesia with   64, 65
  longevity of   68, 69
  nasojugal groove   97, 99
  nasolabial grooves   66
  post-injection instructions   68, 69
  reversibility of   65–66
  selection of   65
  tear troughs   66, 67
  temporal hollows   96–97
  vertical lip lines   37
Hylaform   50

i

immunogenicity   22
Incobotulinum toxin A   20, 21, 75, 76
indirect browlift   35
injection (cosmetic fillers)   64–65, 91–99
  calcium hydroxylapatite   55, 73–74
  ease of use   53–55
  fine lines   92
  glabella   68
  hyaluronic acid   64–65
  labiomandibular groove   93, 94
  labiomental groove   93–95
  lips   66, 97, 98
  melolabial groove   92–93
  midface volumization   94–96
  nasojugal groove   97–99
  nasolabial grooves   66
  post-injection instructions   68
  pre jowl sulcus   93, 94

injection (cosmetic fillers) (*cont'd*)
  tear troughs   67
  temporal hollows   96–97
  wisdom concerning   91–92
injection (neurotoxins)
  brow asymmetry correction   36
  bunny lines   36, 83
  chin dimpling   37–38, 85, 86
  crow's feet   34
  depressor anguili oris   83, 84
  downward-turned commissures of
    mouth   38–39
  forehead   32, 80–81
  glabellar   31, 78–80
  indirect browlift   35
  levator labil superioris alaeque
    nasi   84–85
  lip lengthening   39
  masseter hypertrophy   86–87
  minimizing negative effects of   77–78
  perioral   83, 84
  periorbital   81–82
  platysmal bands   40, 85, 86
  tips for   29–30
  vertical lip lines   37
Instagram   109
intellectual property   110
Internet marketing   103, 110
Isolagen   51, 54

j
jawline   12–13
jowls   2, 13
Juvéderm   64, 66, 68, 92, 93, 96

l
labiomandibular groove   93, 94
labiomental groove   93–95
levator anguli oris (LAO)   6, 7
levator anguli superioris alequea nasi   6, 7
levator labii superioris   6, 7
levator labii superioris alaeque nasi   84–85
lid ptosis   32
ligamentous structures   8–11
linear threading   91–92
LinkedIn   110
lips
  in aging   12, 13
  and CaHA use   72, 73

  fillers for   97, 98
  hyaluronic acid fillers for   66, 67
  lengthening, BoNTA for   39
  muscles related to   6
  neurotoxin injections around   83–85
local anesthesia   64, 65, 73
longevity, of hyaluronic acid fillers   68, 69

m
mandibular ligament   9
marketing   103, 104, 108–111
masseter hypertrophy treatment   86–87
masseteric cutaneous ligaments   9
McGregor's patch   9
melolabial folds   12
melolabial groove   92–93
mentalis muscle   6, 7
microlipoinjection   48
midface
  aging of   12
  ligamentous structures   9
  muscles   6, 7
  volumization in   94–96
mimetic muscles   4–7
minimally-invasive procedures (MIPs)   10,
    13–15, 47
muscles
  mimetic   4–7
  in perioral, nasal, and eyebrow
    regions   2
  SMAS and   3, 5
  of upper face   30

n
nasalis muscle   6, 7
nasojugal groove   97–99
nasolabial fat compartment   2, 8
nasolabial folds   12, 13, 72
nasolabial grooves   66
needles. *See* syringe and needle choices
neurotoxins   19–43
  botulinum neurotoxin A   19–43
  botulinum neurotoxins   19–22
  complications   87–88
  injection techniques   77–87
  preparation and storage   75–76
  syringe and needle choices   76–77
  wisdom in use of   75
nodules   99, 100

Non-Animal Stabilized Hyaluronic Acid
    (NASHA)   64
non-autologous cosmetic fillers   48–51
  bovine collagen   49
  calcium hydroxylapatite   50–51
  dextran beads in hyaluronic acid   50
  hyaluronic acid   50
  poly-L-lactic acid   50
  polymethylmethacrylate   49–50
  polyoxyethylene and
    polyoxypropylene   51
  polytetrafluoroethylene   51
  polyvinyl microspheres suspended in
    polyacrylamide   51
  porcine collagen   49
  silicones   49
  See also specific fillers
non-autologous facial fillers   48–51
nonbiodegradable facial fillers   53, 54. *See
    also specific fillers*
non-reactivity, to BoNTA   22
nonsurgical rhinoplasty   73–74

o

Oculinum   19
Onabotulinum toxin A   20, 21, 75, 76,
    80, 81
online ads   108
orbicularis oculi muscle   6, 7
orbicularis oris muscle   6, 7
orbicularis retaining ligament (ORL)   9
orbicularis-temporal ligament   9
orbital fat   3
overcorrection   99–100

p

paraffin injections   48–49, 53, 54
parotid cutaneous ligament   9–10
patient consultation   24–25, 72, 73
patient evaluation   13–16
  selection and assessment   14–15
  treatment sequencing   15, 16
patient preparation   28–30
perioral region
  in aging   12
  downward-turned commissures of
    mouth   38–39
  excessive chin dimpling   37–38
  lip lengthening   39

  neurotoxin injections in   83, 84
  platysmal bands   39–41
  use of BoNTA in   36–39
  vertical lip lines   36–37
periorbital region
  in aging   11, 12
  ligamentous structures   9
  neurotoxin injections in   81–82
periosteum   1
Perlane   64
permanent fillers   78
photo aging   15
Pinterest   110
Plasmagel   51, 54, 57
platysma   6, 7
platysmal bands   13, 39–41, 85, 86
poly-L-lactic acid   50, 52, 53, 55, 57, 95, 96
polymethylmethacrylate (PMMA)   49–50,
    54, 55, 57, 60
polyoxyethylene and
    polyoxypropylene   51, 54, 61
polytetrafluoroethylene (PTFE)   51, 53,
    54, 60
polyvinyl microspheres suspended in
    polyacrylamide   51, 54, 55, 60
porcine collagen   49, 52, 53
pre jowl sulcus   93, 94
print marketing   104
procerus   5–7
promotion strategy, for practice   103–104
providers of BoNTA treatments   25–26

r

Radiesse   71–74, 92–94, 100
Restylane   63, 64, 92–94, 96, 97
retaining ligaments   8–10
retro-orbicularis fat (ROOF)   8
reversibility, of HA fillers   65–66
risorius muscle   6, 7
Ristow-space   8

s

Sculptra   95–96, 100
Search Engine Optimization
    (SEO)   107–108
serial puncture   91, 92
silicone fillers   49, 53, 54, 60
skin, facial   1–2, 11
SMAS fusion zones   10

social media marketing   108–110
social media protections   110
storage and preparation of
        neurotoxins   26–28, 75–76
subcutaneous fat   1–3, 7–8
subdermal vessels   10
sub-orbicularis oculi fat (SOOF)   8
superficial fat compartments   2–3, 10
superficial musculo-aponeurotic system
        (SMAS)   1–5
superficial temporal fat pad   8
synthetic facial fillers   53
syringe and needle choices
    for CaHA injections   73
    for fat aspiration   54
    for fillers   54, 55, 92
    for neurotoxins   28, 76–77

t

tear troughs   66, 67, 72, 73
temporal hollows   96–97
temporal region
    facial fasciae and   4
    subcutaneous fat of   3
temporoparietal fascia   4
tissue descent   11–12
treatment sequencing   15, 16
Twitter   109
Tyndall effect   65, 100

u
upper face
    BoNTA treatments   30–36
    crow's feet treatment   32, 34–35
    diffusion of product in   42
    forehead treatments   32–34

glabella treatment   30–32
ligamentous structures   9
muscles   5–7, 9, 30

v
vascular compromise   100–102
vertical lip lines   36, 37, 83, 84
Vitrase   66, 68, 69
Volbella   92
Vollure   92
Voluma   65, 68, 94

w
website design   104–108
    choosing designers   104–106
    companies specializing in   114
    creating the website   106–107
    online ads   108
    Search Engine Optimization
        107–108
wrinkles, Glogau classification of   15

x
xenograft facial fillers   53
Xeomin   20–22, 27–28, 30, 76

y
YouTube   109–110

z
zones of fixation   9, 10
Zyderm   49, 63
zygomatic ligaments   9
zygomaticus major   6, 7
zygomaticus minor   6, 7
Zyplast   49, 63